Vegan Buddha Bowls

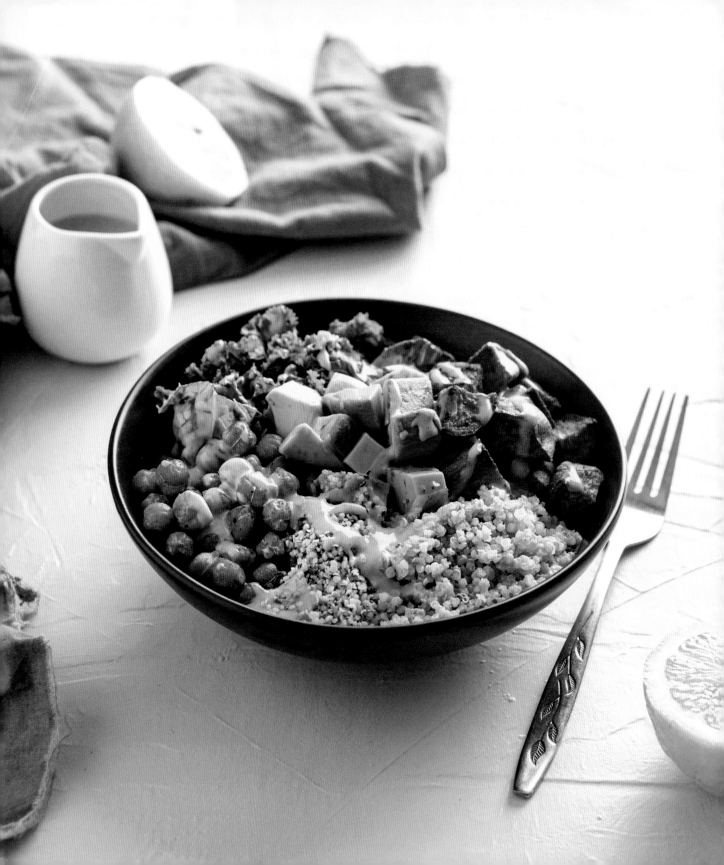

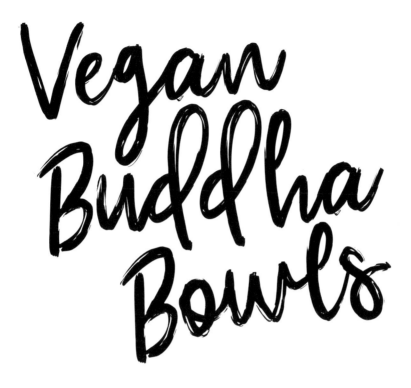

Vegan Buddha Bowls

EASY, HEALTHY RECIPES TO FEEL GREAT
FROM THE INSIDE OUT

Cara Carin Cifelli

CREATOR OF CARA'S KITCHEN

PAGE STREET
PUBLISHING CO.

PAGE STREET
PUBLISHING CO.

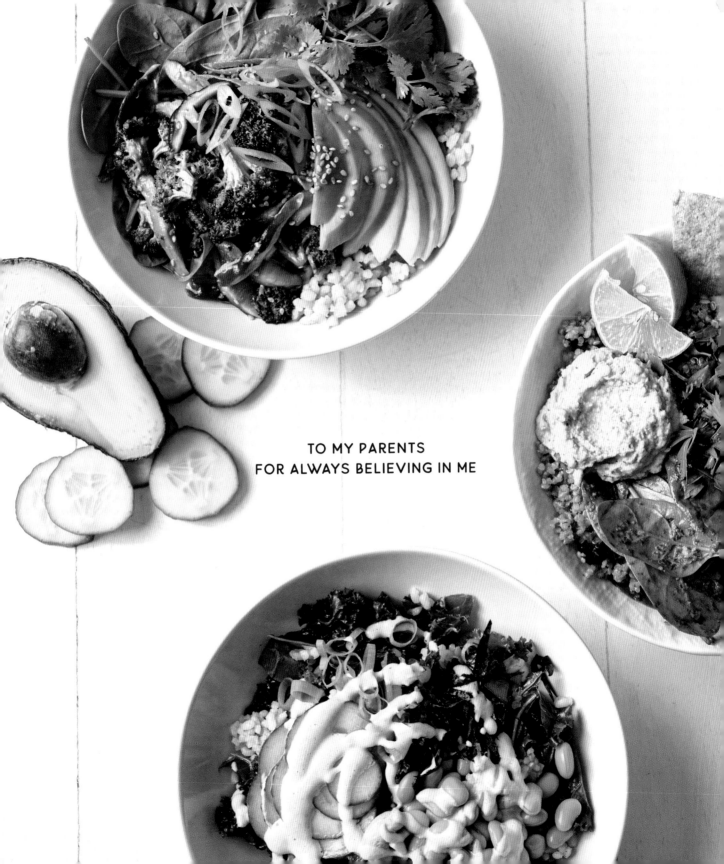

TO MY PARENTS
FOR ALWAYS BELIEVING IN ME

Contents

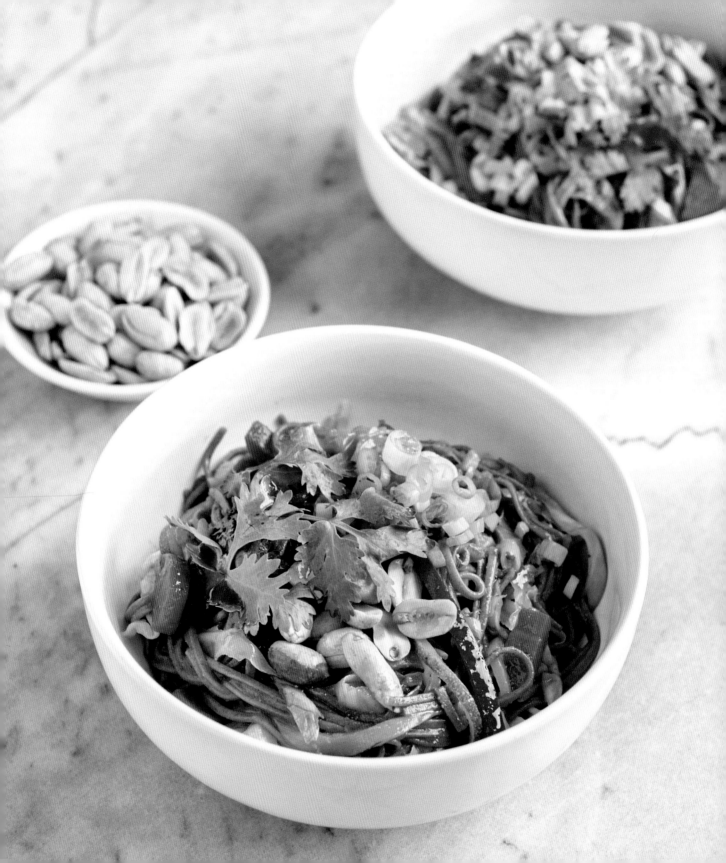

Introduction

One of my favorite quotes from Steve Jobs is, "You can't connect the dots looking forward; you can only connect them looking backward. So you have to trust that the dots will somehow connect in your future. You have to trust in something—your gut, destiny, life, karma, whatever. This approach has never let me down, and it has made all the difference in my life."

When I look back at all the dots in my past that led me to this point, writing this cookbook, I am somewhat in awe. While it all makes sense—each dot was necessary, they do in fact connect—I am no less surprised to be here now. I feel grateful, humbled, excited, all of that, and yet, I haven't always felt that way about life . . . or food, for that matter.

While growing up, I had a very normal, intuitive relationship with food and naturally ate a variety of things in a balanced way. My mom cooked for us, but we were by no means a foodie household. She cooked out of necessity, not passion, so I was never in the kitchen learning from her and I don't have any secret family recipes passed down and shared within the pages of this book.

To be honest, for so much of my childhood, we ate at fast-food restaurants or I was microwaving a frozen pizza pocket for dinner. There is nothing wrong with this, nor am I trying to share it in a negative light. Rather, my point is that I didn't grow up loving food or knowing how to cook—food was just food; it was sort of no big deal.

That all began to shift around age fourteen or fifteen, when I became increasingly aware of the pressure and importance our society places on us to be thin. I internalized the importance of looking a certain way from every possible avenue, including magazines, TV, friends and the women in my family. It led to me trying my first diet, and over time snowballed into a big, hairy problem known as an eating disorder, and it took over my life, just as it does the lives of so many.

I struggled with my relationship with food, which was also a reflection of the relationship I had with myself for ten years. And it made everyday life difficult. Things like birthday parties or going out to eat caused me stress and anxiety. Being present with my family and friends on holidays seemed impossible as I was always freaking out about the food, about whether I would binge or people would be judging me for what I looked like. With each passing day when I felt I had failed with food, my self-worth and self-esteem took a hit. Until, I hit rock bottom.

I've come to believe that rock bottom, even as painful as it is, is a beautiful place from which you can rebuild your life. Getting there was truly the darkest experience I've ever had, and yet it gave me my brightest light. It's true what they say: The wound is where the light enters.

I started to take recovery seriously and a huge part of that was educating myself about nutrition outside the context of weight loss. Discovering that different foods had different nutrients that could help my body thrive inspired me to eat in a way that dieting and trying to be thin never could. It made food about self-care, not self-control or weight control. By continuing down the rabbit hole of whole food nutrition, I also discovered that I could eat in a way that aligned with my values to take care of the planet and eat locally as much as possible. It changed everything, and it's what inspired me to teach myself how to cook.

Without my eating disorder, I likely never would have had an interest in food or following others' recipes, which ultimately led to me creatively expressing myself by coming up with my own. It's also safe to say that I probably would not have started a food blog, which led to me opening (and then later selling) a restaurant, nor would I have written and published my first book, *Body Wisdom*, and I sure as hell would not have become a health coach helping others heal their relationship with food and their body, too.

You see, all those dots connect. And they are what have led me to this point writing this book full of my creative energy and love for nourishing, plant-based foods. Here you will find some of my favorite body-loving, soul-nourishing Buddha bowl recipes. I've always had a love of eating food from a bowl because there is a comfort element to the way it just holds everything together.

A major bonus about so many of these recipes is that they are great for meal prep. They keep well for days in the refrigerator, which is something that has been important to me. When I go through the effort to shop and cook from scratch, which is regularly, I love having leftovers the next day for lunch. So, whether you prep ahead for the week or simply the next day, you will find directions for storage in the chapter introductions or toward the end of each recipe's instructions, when appropriate.

In addition to storing well, a lot of these bowls are also easy to make without an excess of ingredients. For many of us who work full-time, having something simple, delicious and pretty quick to prepare when you finish up for the day is of supreme value.

Something I've discovered is that delicious food doesn't have to be complicated food, and these recipes attest to that. Something that I've also learned over the years that has helped make my food taste good is to season your food with salt and pepper through the entire cooking process, not just at the end. This will help bring out the flavors of each ingredient and the end result will taste that much better. You will notice that each recipe says to salt to taste, and this is why: You have taste buds, so use them and season to your liking. Also, several recipes will list lemon or lime as a garnish. A fresh squeeze of citrus on top before serving often gives a dish that last little something it needs to really pop!

The last couple of tips I want to add here about these recipes are that several of them require the use of a blender, so I recommend a high-speed one, such as Vitamix. If you do not have one and you are making a recipe using nuts, the soaking time may vary, and I recommend soaking for an additional 30 minutes to an hour to protect your blender. And lastly, several recipes call for rice that is already cooked. The standard measurement rule here is that 1 cup (195 g) of uncooked rice + 2 cups (475 ml) of water or broth = 3 cups (510 g) of cooked rice. Making a bulk batch of rice can help make the Good Karma Bowl (page 14), Sweet Sesame Rice Bowl (page 21), Tangy Tofu Bowl (page 41) and Crowd-Pleasing Curry Bowl (page 33).

I truly hope you enjoy cooking from this book as much as I enjoyed writing it. I hope that making yourself meals from this book is an expression of self-care and leaves you feeling energized and vibrant.

Thank you for allowing me to be a part of your journey through this book.

Xo Cara

Cara Cifelli

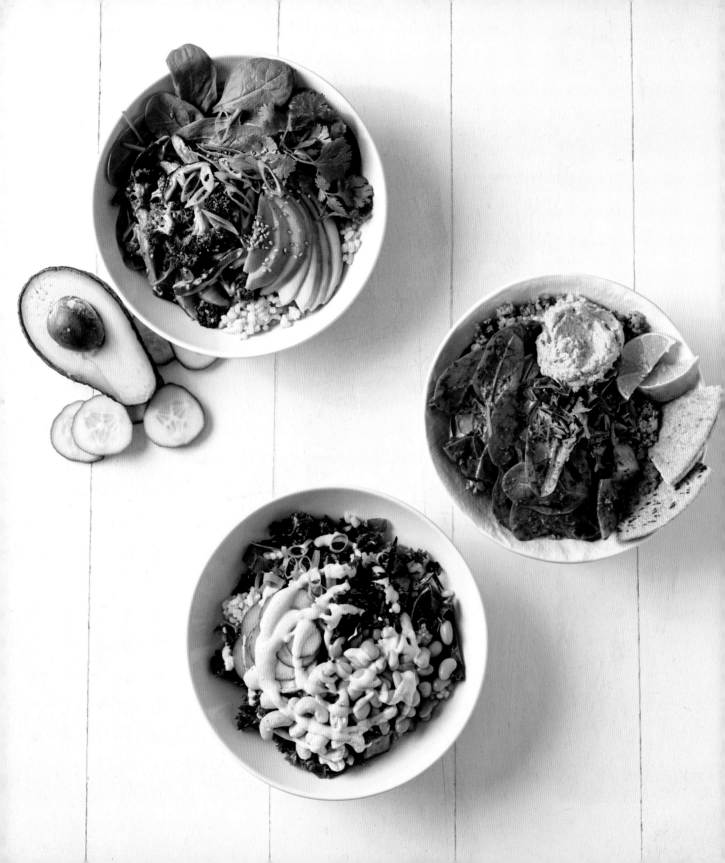

Beautiful, Bountiful Buddha Bowls

I've been a fan of the Buddha bowl from the minute I discovered it. Like any delicious bowl, the recipes in this chapter combine an eclectic mix of ingredients, often with varying textures, flavors and colors to make the whole experience more enjoyable. As a bonus, many of them are also great to make ahead or use for meal prep, too. Although some bowls here have several elements, a key pillar of my style of cooking is keeping things simple (most of the time) without sacrificing flavor. Some of my favorite recipes for that are the Sweet Sesame Rice Bowl (page 21), The Classic Buddha Bowl (page 17), The Green Machine (page 37), The Roasted Veg (page 29) and the Harissa Curry Bowl (page 38). I hope you fall in love with these recipes as much as I have.

Nearly all of these recipes can be made ahead of time. If making ahead for meal prep, simply mix everything as stated, storing the sauce and garnishes separately, if you'd prefer. For the bowl, you can divide it into single servings or store it in one large container for up to one week.

Good Karma Bowl

I love how Buddha bowls allow you to fuse together creative flavor combinations, such as this zippy yet rich ginger tahini on bright crunchy cucumbers, kale and edamame. The grounding rice and sweet potatoes round out the dish and make it a substantial meal. Top it off with seaweed for some umami and cashews for extra crunch, and you have yourself one delicious, filling and soulful Buddha bowl.

--- SERVES 4 ---

BOWL

4 cups (532 g) cubed sweet potato (½" [1.2-cm] cubes])

1 tbsp (15 ml) avocado oil

Pinch of garlic powder

Pink salt

1 cup (119 g) thinly sliced English cucumber

¾ cup (175 ml) water

¼ cup (60 ml) apple cider vinegar

4 cups (268 g) stemmed and chopped curly kale (bite-size pieces)

Juice of 1 lemon

2 tsp (10 ml) olive oil

4 cups (780 g) cooked brown rice

1 cup (155 g) edamame

¼ cup (35 g) salted dry-roasted cashews

¼ cup (28 g) dry-roasted seaweed

1 green onion, thinly sliced

GINGER & GARLIC TAHINI SAUCE

⅔ cup (160 g) tahini

¾ cup (175 ml) water

1 (2" [5-cm]) knob fresh ginger, peeled

4 cloves garlic

1 tbsp (15 ml) honey or pure maple syrup

¼ cup (60 ml) fresh lime juice

½ tsp pink salt, plus more to taste

GARNISHES

Crushed red pepper flakes

Hemp seeds

Pink sauerkraut

Lemon wedges

Preheat the oven to 450°F (230°C). In a bowl, lightly coat the sweet potato with the avocado oil, add the garlic powder and a pinch of pink salt and toss to evenly coat. Lay out in a single layer on a baking sheet and roast in the oven for 13 to 17 minutes, or until crispy and browned on one side. Remove from the oven and set aside.

Meanwhile, in a jar or bowl, combine the cucumber slices, water and vinegar. Add a pinch of salt and mix well. Set aside.

In a large bowl, combine the kale with the lemon juice, olive oil and a pinch of pink salt. Using your hands or a pair of tongs, massage the kale. Set aside.

Make the sauce: In a high-speed blender, combine the tahini, water, ginger, garlic, honey, lime juice and pink salt and blend on high speed until smooth.

Add the rice and sweet potatoes to the kale and mix. Divide among 4 serving bowls. Drain the cucumber, then layer the edamame, cucumber, cashews, seaweed and green onion on top. Add the garnishes and top with the sauce. You may have a little more sauce than you need. If that is the case, simply store the remainder in an airtight container in the fridge for up to a week.

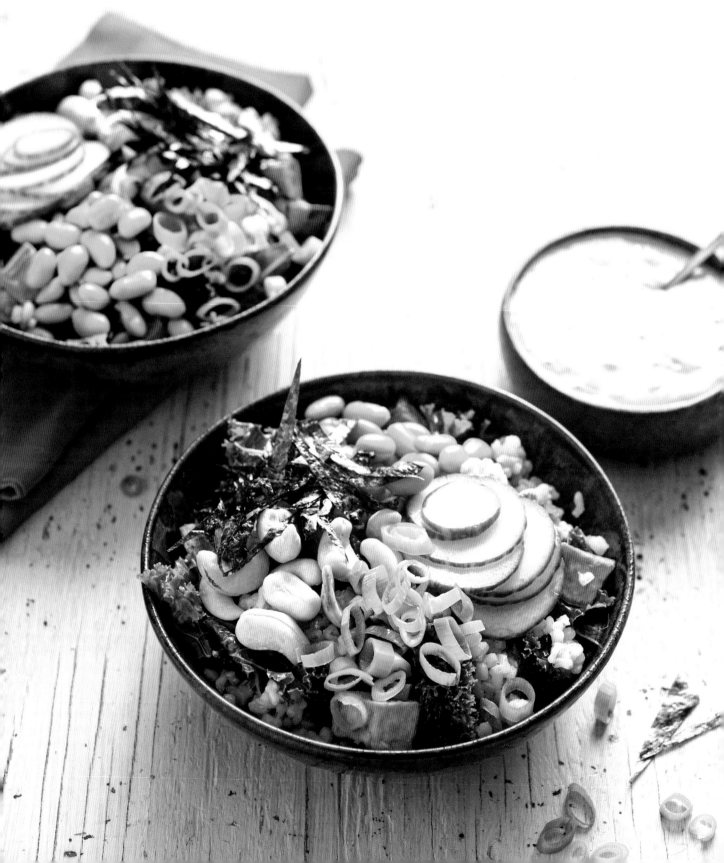

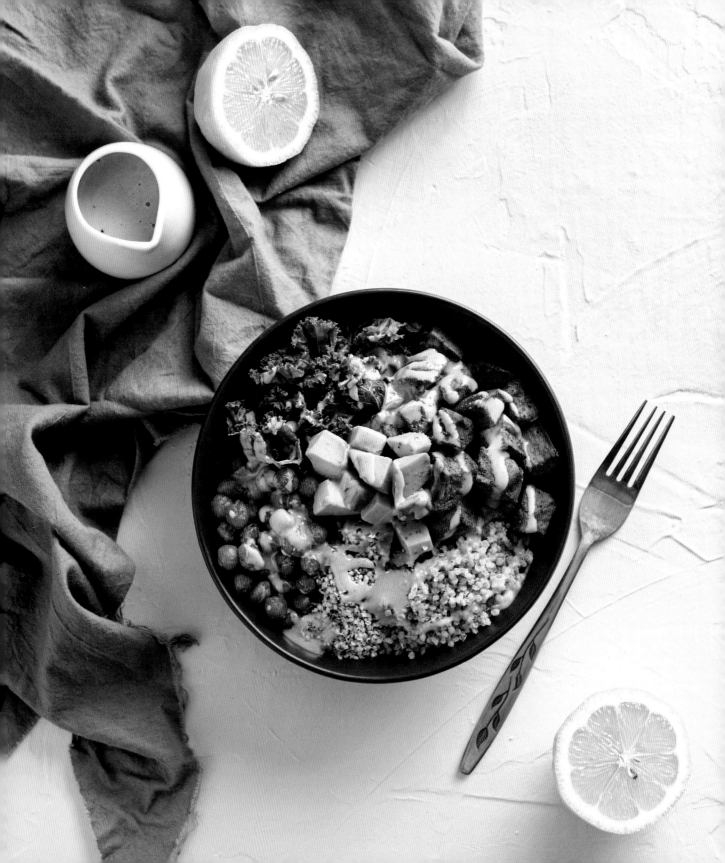

The Classic Buddha Bowl

After years of being on Instagram, I can confidently say this is the OG Buddha bowl. I feel that it is the most classic combination, and with good reason: it's easy to make and it's a freakin' mouth party! Roasting the sweet potatoes brings out their sweetness, which pairs perfectly with the spiced garbanzo beans. The quinoa makes it extra filling and what would a Buddha bowl be without an avocado? Everything is married together with a delicious maple tahini drizzle.

SERVES 2

SAUCE

½ cup (120 g) tahini

⅓ cup (80 ml) water

2 tbsp (30 ml) pure maple syrup

2 cloves garlic, grated (preferred) or minced

2 tbsp (30 ml) lemon juice

Salt and freshly ground black pepper

BOWL

4 cups (532 g) cubed sweet potato (¾" [2-cm] cubes)

1 tbsp (14 g) coconut oil

1 tsp garlic powder, divided

½ tsp ground cumin, divided

½ tsp smoked paprika, divided

Salt and freshly ground black pepper

1 (15-oz [425-g]) can garbanzo beans, drained and rinsed

2 cups (370 g) cooked white quinoa

2 cups (134 g) tightly packed, chopped steamed kale

GARNISHES

Avocado

Fresh lemon juice

Hemp seeds

Make the sauce: In a small bowl, whisk together the tahini, water, maple syrup, garlic, lemon juice and salt and pepper to taste. Set aside.

Preheat the oven to 450°F (230°C).

Make the veggies: In a bowl, toss together the sweet potato, coconut oil, ½ teaspoon of the garlic powder and ¼ teaspoon each of the cumin and smoked paprika. Season with salt and pepper to taste. Lay out in an even layer on a baking sheet, leaving some room on one side to later add the garbanzo beans. Roast in the oven for 8 to 10 minutes, then remove from the oven.

Add the garbanzo beans to the space you left for them and toss them with the remaining ½ teaspoon of garlic powder and remaining ¼ teaspoon each of cumin and smoked paprika. Return the pan to the oven and roast for another 8 to 10 minutes, or until the sweet potatoes are fork-tender.

Build your bowls by dividing the quinoa, kale, sweet potatoes and garbanzo beans between 2 serving bowls. Add the sauce to each bowl and garnish with avocado, lemon juice and hemp seeds. Serve immediately. If making ahead of time for meal prep, I recommend waiting to add the avocado until ready to serve.

The Humble Bowl

This recipe features creamy white beans with crunchy roasted veggies and sweet fresh herbs. It's an unusual combination that is tied together perfectly with a bright shallot vinaigrette that will keep you coming back for more. It is inspired by the talented Samin Nosrat, whose passion for food and cooking is electric and contagious. Her enthusiasm gets you excited about eating. And as someone who struggled with an eating disorder, I know that eating can sometimes be a tremendously scary feat. But she infuses so much joy and love into all she creates, it leaves you with a sense of what's possible in your relationship with food. One bite of this recipe and you will understand the pleasure of eating.

————————————————————— SERVES 2 —————————————————————

BEANS

1 tbsp (14 g) coconut oil

½ cup (80 g) diced onion

2 cloves garlic, minced

Salt

1 cup (225 g) dried large white lima beans

5 cups (1.2 L) water

1 bay leaf

Freshly ground black pepper

VEGGIES

3 cups (213 g) broccoli florets

2 cups (176 g) Brussels sprouts, halved

1 large head cauliflower, chopped into florets

6 carrots, sliced into quarters lengthwise

3 tbsp (45 ml) melted coconut oil

2 tsp (6 g) garlic powder

Salt and freshly ground black pepper

SHALLOT VINAIGRETTE

1 shallot, diced

¼ cup (60 ml) red wine vinegar

½ cup (120 ml) olive oil

1 tsp za'atar

1 tsp garlic powder

Salt and freshly ground black pepper

TO SERVE

Avocado oil

Za'atar

1 cup (60 g) loosely packed roughly chopped fresh parsley

1 cup (40 g) loosely packed roughly chopped fresh cilantro

½ cup (20 g) loosely packed roughly chopped fresh mint

Make the beans: In a medium-sized soup pot, melt the coconut oil over medium heat. Once hot, add the onion and cook for 3 to 5 minutes, then add the garlic, season generously with salt and, stirring constantly, cook for another 30 seconds. Meanwhile, rinse and drain the beans, then add them to the pot. Add the water and bay leaf and season again with a big pinch of salt and pepper. Bring to a boil and boil, uncovered, for 10 minutes. Cover, lower the heat to a simmer, then cook for 45 minutes to 1 hour, or until cooked through and fork-tender. Once the beans are cooked through, drain the water, discard the bay leaf and set the beans aside.

While the beans cook, make the vegetables: Preheat the oven to 450°F (230°C).

Lay out the broccoli, Brussels sprouts, cauliflower and carrots in a single layer on 1 or 2 baking sheets, giving them room to breathe. Drizzle with the coconut oil and toss them to coat on all sides. Season with the garlic powder and salt and pepper to taste. Roast in the oven, stirring once midway through the roasting time, for 15 to 25 minutes, or until tender and the edges are golden brown. Remove from the oven and set aside.

Meanwhile, make the vinaigrette: In a small bowl, combine the shallot and vinegar and let marinate for 30 minutes, stirring occasionally. Then, whisk in the olive oil, add the za'atar and garlic powder and season generously with salt and pepper.

Assemble the dish: Lay out the vegetables on a large serving tray or plate and cover with half of the dressing. Drizzle with avocado oil to taste and sprinkle with za'atar. Add the beans and fresh herbs, then cover with the remaining dressing. Serve immediately.

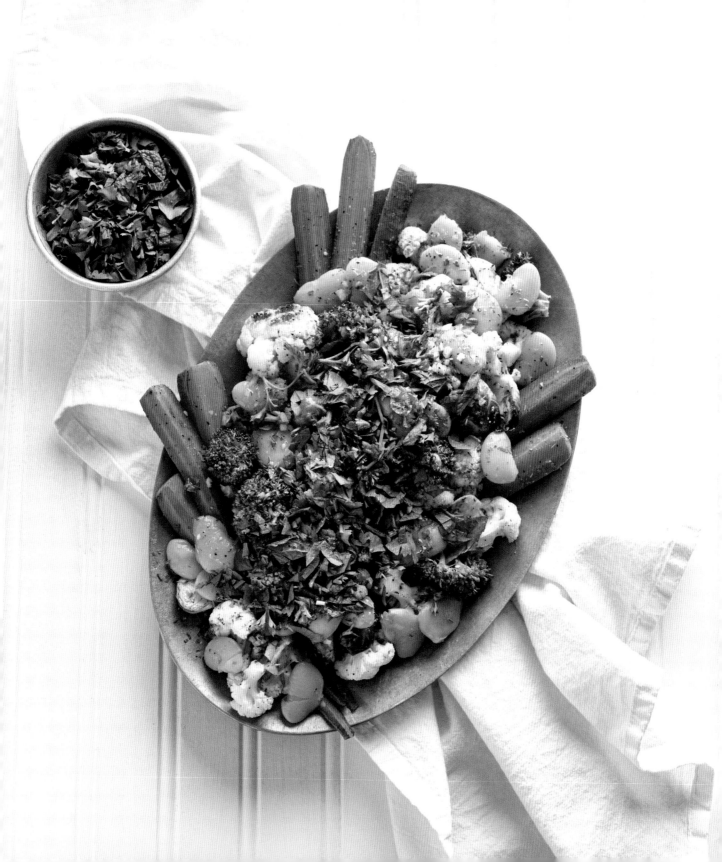

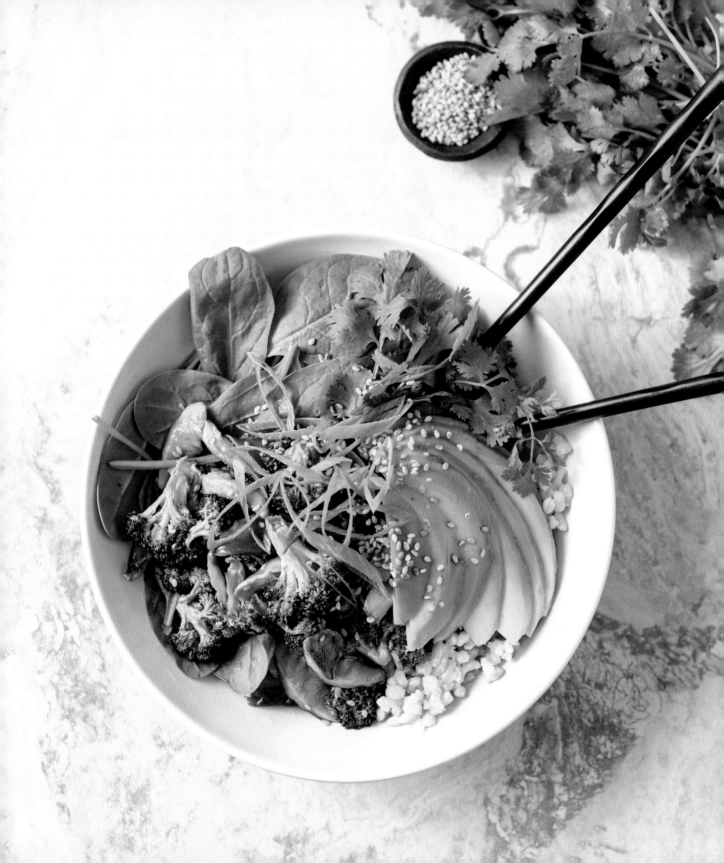

Sweet Sesame Rice Bowl

This is one of those bowls that might seem unassuming at first glance, but with the creamy and slightly sweet coconut rice, it's an elevated take on the traditional veggie and rice bowls you might be used to. It combines sweet broccoli with savory shiitake mushrooms and is tied together perfectly with a honey-sesame sauce that is finger-licking good. I added some spinach for an extra-nutritious kick and rich avocado because . . . you know, avocado. This just might be your new favorite weeknight meal.

--- SERVES 2 ---

RICE

1 cup (190 g) uncooked brown jasmine rice

1 cup (240 ml) full-fat coconut milk

1¼ cups (295 ml) water

½ tsp salt

HONEY-SESAME SAUCE

¼ cup (60 ml) soy sauce or tamari

¼ cup (60 ml) rice vinegar

¼ cup (60 ml) water

1 tbsp (8 g) arrowroot starch

¼ cup (60 ml) honey

2 tsp (10 ml) toasted sesame oil

2 tsp (6 g) sesame seeds

VEGGIES

6 cups (426 g) chopped broccoli florets

3 tbsp (45 ml) melted coconut oil, divided

Salt and freshly ground black pepper

7 oz (198 g) shiitake mushrooms, sliced

2 cups (65 g) tightly packed fresh baby spinach

GARNISHES

1 ripe avocado, sliced

Green onion

Fresh cilantro

Sesame seeds

Preheat the oven to 450°F (230°C).

Make the rice: In a small soup pot, combine the rice, coconut milk, water and salt. Bring to a boil, cover, lower the heat to a simmer and cook for 25 to 30 minutes, or until all the moisture has been absorbed.

Meanwhile, make the sauce: In a small bowl, whisk together the soy sauce, vinegar, water, arrowroot, honey, sesame oil and sesame seeds. Set aside.

While the rice cooks, also make the veggies: In a bowl, evenly coat the broccoli florets with 1½ tablespoons (22 ml) of the coconut oil, season with salt and pepper, then lay out in a single layer on a baking sheet. Roast in the oven for 8 to 9 minutes.

In a large skillet, heat the remaining 1½ tablespoons (23 ml) of coconut oil over medium heat. Once hot, add the mushrooms and cook for 5 minutes, then add ¼ cup (60 ml) of the sauce and cook, stirring continuously, until almost absorbed, about 1 to 2 minutes. Continue to cook for another 2 to 3 minutes, then add the broccoli to the pan along with another ¼ cup (60 ml) of the sauce. Cook, stirring continuously, until the sauce is absorbed, 3 to 5 minutes. Turn off the heat.

To make the bowls, divide the rice, spinach and veggies between 2 serving bowls. Cover with the remaining sauce, then garnish with sliced avocado, green onion, cilantro and sesame seeds. Dig in!

Pesto Party Bowl

If I had to choose a favorite cuisine, it would be Mediterranean, hands down. The ingredients are often easy to find, fairly affordable and always full of flavor. If I still worked at an office, this would be one of my favorite recipes to take along for lunch, because the quinoa salad is easy to make and keeps well in the fridge for days. With a handful of fresh spinach, a dollop of delicious basil pesto and a side of pita and hummus, you have yourself anything but a sad desk lunch. It's filling, tasty and easy to make, truly a winning combination in my book!

SERVES 4

QUINOA

1½ cups (260 g) dried white quinoa

2 to 3 cloves garlic, grated (preferred) or minced

3 cups (710 ml) vegetable broth

BASIL PESTO

½ cup (67 g) pine nuts

4 cloves garlic

2 tbsp (16 g) nutritional yeast

6 cups (240 g) lightly packed fresh basil leaves

¼ cup (60 ml) fresh lemon juice

1 tsp salt

⅔ cup (160 ml) olive oil

BOWL

½ cup (55 g) diced oil-packed sun-dried tomatoes (see Notes)

½ cup (50 g) pitted and diced Kalamata olives

¾ cup (101 g) chopped cucumber (½" [1.3-cm] pieces)

2 green onions, sliced

6 oz (170 g) baby spinach

FOR SERVING & GARNISHES

Hummus

Pita bread

Chopped fresh parsley

Fresh lemon juice (optional)

Olive oil, for drizzling

In a small soup pot, combine the quinoa, garlic and vegetable broth. Bring to a boil over high heat, cover, then lower the heat to low. Simmer until all the liquid is absorbed, 12 to 14 minutes. Fluff with a fork and set aside to cool down for 10 minutes.

While the quinoa cooks, make the basil pesto: In a food processor, combine the pine nuts, garlic, nutritional yeast, basil, lemon juice and salt. Pulse in 3-second bursts for a total of 30 to 45 seconds, or until everything is finely diced but not turned into a paste. Then, with the processor on low speed, slowly drizzle in the olive oil through the center of the lid until a thick, slightly chunky paste is formed. Set aside the pesto while finishing up the rest of the dish.

Once the quinoa has cooled down, transfer it to a medium-sized bowl. Add the sun-dried tomatoes, olives, cucumber, green onion and ⅓ cup (87 g) of the basil pesto. Mix well to evenly combine. Divide the quinoa among 4 serving bowls.

Then, in the same bowl used for the quinoa, combine the spinach and ⅓ cup (87 g) of basil pesto. Toss to evenly coat. Divide the spinach mixture equally among the 4 serving bowls.

Add a dollop of hummus to each bowl and serve with pita bread. Add parsley, a spritz of lemon juice (if desired) and a drizzle of olive oil and serve.

Notes: *You will likely have more pesto than you need, so save some for toasts or pasta. The remainder will keep well in an airtight container in the fridge for up to a week.*

If desired, you can substitute diced cherry tomatoes for the sun-dried, for a fresher vibe.

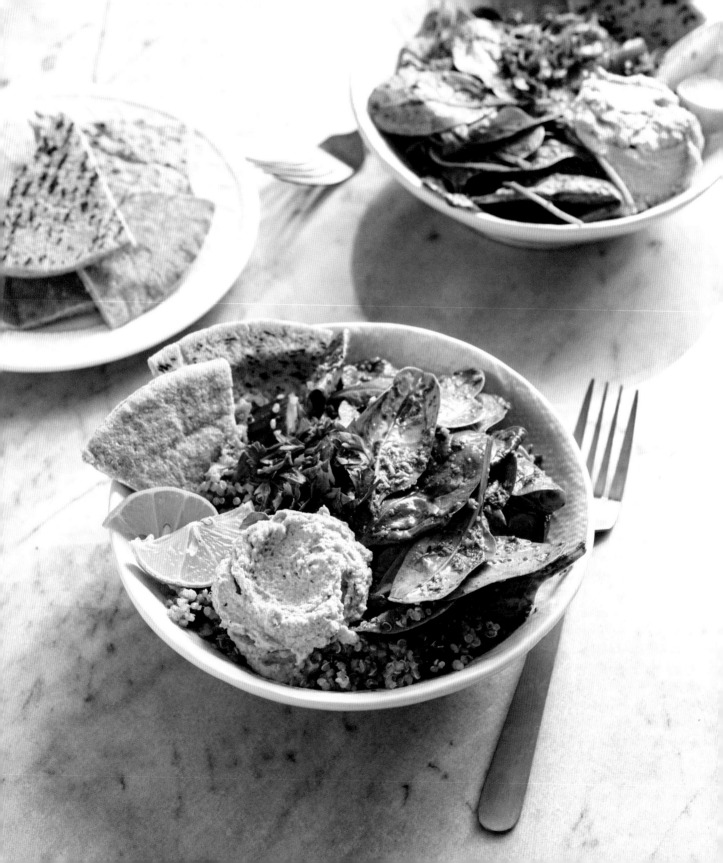

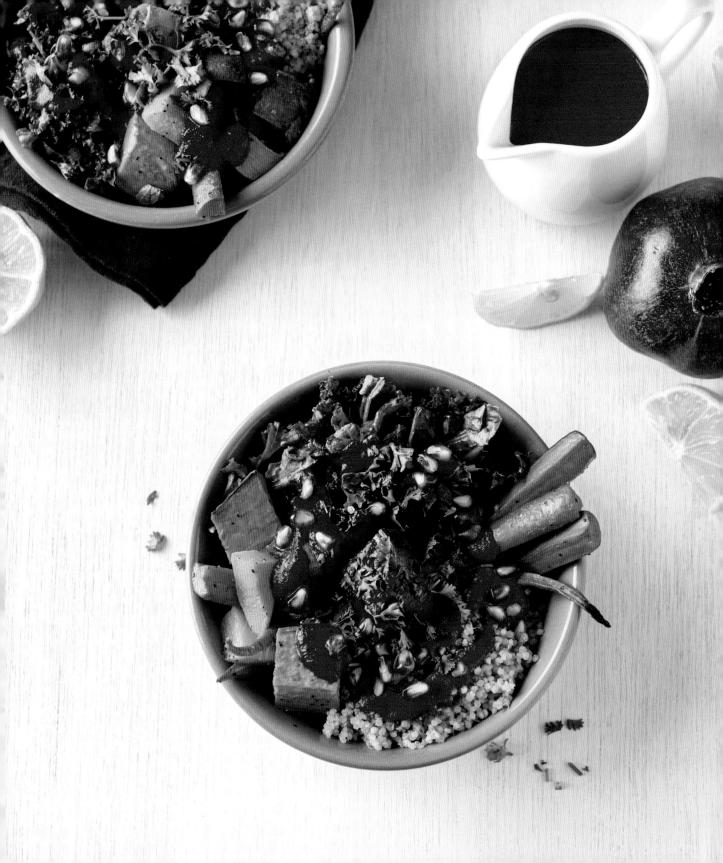

Beetroot Beauty Bowl

There is something fun about saying "beetroot tahini," isn't there? While growing up, I was not a fan of beets, but as I started to enjoy all vegetables more and realized that how you prepare them massively changes their flavor, they grew on me. This bowl features the best of grounding fall produce— butternut squash, carrots, sweet potatoes and beets—all of which I would argue are best when roasted. This caramelizes their sugars, bringing out their natural sweetness. They are perfectly balanced by the bitter kale, bright lemon juice and pomegranate seeds and the rich beetroot tahini. And the addition of quinoa makes this a well-rounded, soulful meal.

SERVES 4

VEGGIES

3 cups (420 g) cubed butternut squash (1" [2.5-cm] cubes)

3 cups (400 g) cubed sweet potato (1" [2.5-cm] cubes)

5 carrots, sliced into quarters, lengthwise

3 tbsp (45 ml) melted coconut oil

2 tbsp (13 g) curry powder (Indian variety with turmeric)

Salt and freshly ground black pepper

4 cups (268 g) chopped kale

Juice of ½ to 1 lemon

1 to 2 tsp (5 to 10 ml) olive oil

BEETROOT TAHINI

1 cup (224 g) cubed roasted red beet, (½" [1.2-cm] cubes)

½ cup (120 ml) water

¼ cup (60 g) tahini

2 cloves garlic

2 tbsp (30 ml) fresh lemon juice

1½ tbsp (22 ml) honey

Salt and freshly ground black pepper

BOWL

2 cups (340 g) cooked white quinoa

¼ cup (56 g) pomegranate seeds (see Note)

Chopped fresh parsley or cilantro

Preheat the oven to 450°F (230°C).

Make the vegetables: In a bowl, toss the butternut squash, sweet potatoes and carrots with the melted coconut oil, curry powder and salt and pepper to taste. If you are roasting the beet from scratch (for the tahini), add it in this step. Cut the beet into small cubes and add it to the tossed vegetables. Lay out the vegetable mixture on a baking sheet and roast in the oven for 15 to 25 minutes, or until everything is fork-tender. Remove from the oven and set aside.

In a large bowl, combine the chopped kale with the lemon juice, salt to taste and olive oil. Using your hands or a pair of tongs, massage the kale for 1 to 2 minutes. Set aside.

Make the beetroot tahini: In a high-speed blender, combine the roasted beet, water, tahini, garlic, lemon juice, honey and salt and pepper to taste. Blend on high speed until smooth. Taste and see whether you want to adjust any of the seasonings.

Build your bowls by dividing the quinoa, kale, veggies and sauce among 4 serving bowls. Top with the pomegranate seeds and fresh parsley. Serve immediately.

Note: *To save time, you could buy ready-to-use pomegranate seeds instead of removing them from the fruit on your own. It can truly be a tedious, time-consuming task!*

Tropical Poke Bowls

I remember the first time I made this recipe. I was the chef at a women's transformational retreat in Joshua Tree, California, and this was the most popular dish from the weekend, so I knew I had to make sure it made its way into the cookbook. Not only is it a filling and well-rounded bowl, it's also an incredibly refreshing dish. The watermelon and mango add such a juicy kick to the grounding quinoa and tofu. The cucumber and cabbage add necessary crunch that is balanced out by the creamy avocado. Topped off with a luxurious drizzle of a tangy lime–almond butter sauce, this will be on high rotation during the summer months!

--- SERVES 4 ---

TANGY LIME–ALMOND BUTTER SAUCE

¾ cup (195 g) almond butter

½ cup (120 ml) water

1 (½" [1.2-cm]) knob fresh ginger, peeled

3 tbsp (45 ml) fresh lime juice, plus more to taste

2 tsp (10 ml) soy sauce or tamari

2 tsp (10 ml) pure maple syrup

¼ tsp garlic powder

⅛ tsp cayenne pepper

BOWL

1 cup (173 g) uncooked white quinoa

2 cups (475 ml) vegetable broth

1 (15.5-oz [439-g]) package extra-firm tofu

2 tbsp (28 g) coconut oil

1 tsp garlic powder

½ tsp curry powder

Salt

1 medium-sized cabbage, shredded

1 English cucumber, thinly sliced

1 ripe mango, cut into ½" (1.2-cm) cubes

4 cups (610 g) cubed watermelon (½" [1.2-cm] cubes)

1 ripe avocado, sliced

GARNISHES

Fresh cilantro

Green onion

Hemp seeds

Crushed red pepper flakes

Lime wedges

Make the sauce: In a blender, combine the almond butter, water, ginger, lime juice, soy sauce, maple syrup, garlic powder and cayenne. Blend on high speed until smooth. Set aside.

Make the quinoa and tofu for the bowl: In a small saucepan, combine the quinoa and vegetable broth. Bring to a boil, then cover and lower the heat to a simmer. Cook until all the liquid is absorbed, about 12 minutes, then remove from the heat and set aside.

While the quinoa cooks, drain the water from the tofu and wrap it in a clean dish towel. Firmly press down to remove as much water as possible, then cut into ½-inch (1.2-cm) cubes. In a medium-sized saucepan, melt the coconut oil over medium heat. Once hot, add the tofu and cook for 8 minutes, stirring every 2 minutes. Then, add the garlic powder and curry powder. Toss to evenly coat, add salt to taste and remove from the heat.

Layer the cabbage, quinoa, tofu, cucumber, mango, watermelon and avocado equally among 4 serving bowls and then toss or leave them layered, as you desire. Top each bowl with the sauce and garnish with the cilantro, green onion, hemp seeds, red pepper flakes and lime wedges. Serve immediately.

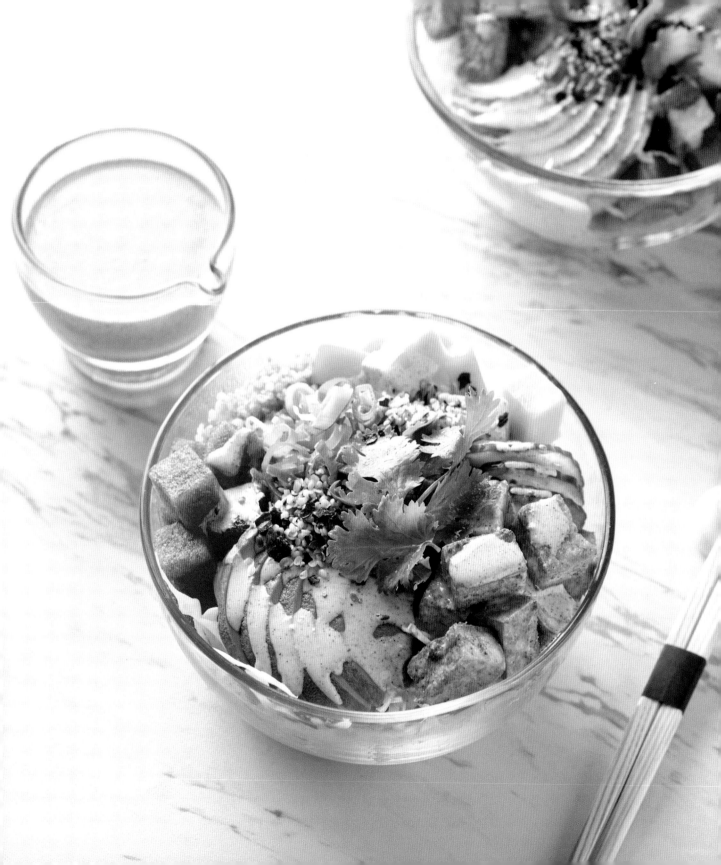

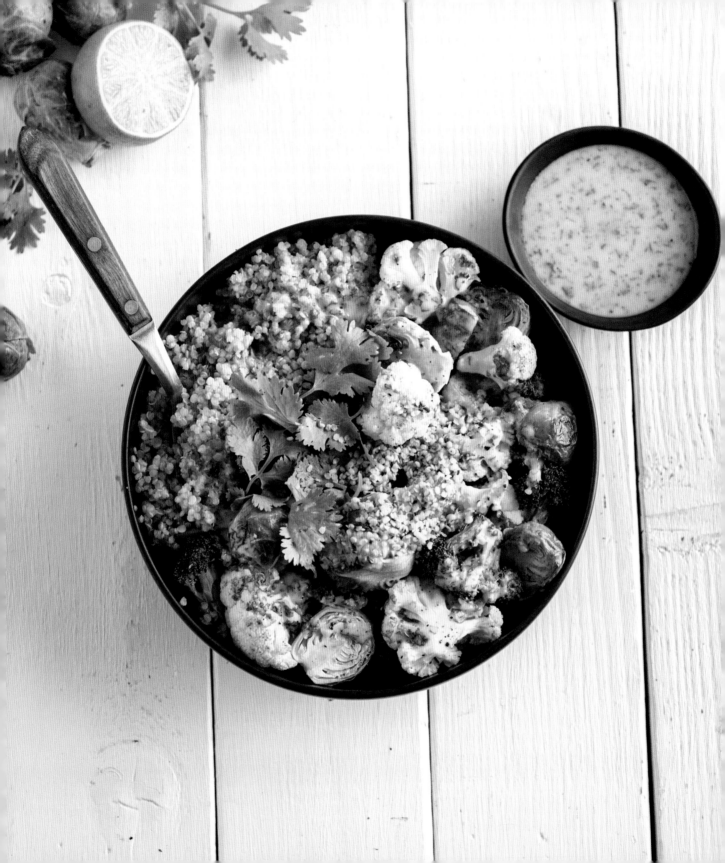

The Roasted Veg

This bowl—so simple, so good—pretty much sums up my food philosophy. The herbaceous yet sweet creamy tahini sauce is easy to make and beautifully coats the roasted cruciferous veggies. The quinoa makes it more substantial and filling. Perfect for a quick and nutritious weeknight meal.

————————————————————— SERVES 2 —————————————————————

BOWL

1 cup (173 g) uncooked white quinoa

2 cups (475 ml) vegetable broth

1 medium-sized cauliflower, cut into florets

4 carrots, sliced into quarters lengthwise

3 cups (213 g) broccoli florets

3 cups (264 g) halved Brussels sprouts

2 tbsp (30 ml) avocado oil

Salt and freshly ground black pepper

CILANTRO TAHINI SAUCE

1 cup (40 g) finely chopped fresh cilantro leaves

½ cup (120 ml) avocado oil

¼ cup (60 ml) lime juice

3 tbsp (45 ml) apple cider vinegar

¼ cup (60 g) tahini

2 tbsp (30 ml) maple syrup

1 to 2 cloves garlic, minced

Salt and freshly ground black pepper

GARNISHES

Hemp seeds

Fresh cilantro

Preheat the oven to 450°F (230°C).

In a small saucepan, combine the quinoa and vegetable broth. Bring to a boil, cover, then lower the heat to a simmer. Cook for 10 to 12 minutes, or until all the liquid is absorbed. Set aside.

Lay out the cauliflower, carrots, broccoli and Brussels sprouts in a single layer on 1 or 2 baking sheets. Add the avocado oil and toss to coat. Season with salt and pepper to taste. Roast in the oven for 15 to 18 minutes, or until golden brown on one side. Remove from the oven and set aside.

While the quinoa and veggies cook, make the sauce: In a small bowl, whisk together the cilantro, avocado oil, lime juice, vinegar, tahini, maple syrup, garlic and salt and pepper to taste.

Divide the quinoa and vegetables equally between 2 serving bowls, then divide the sauce between the bowls. Garnish with hemp seeds and cilantro and serve.

Southern Comfort Bowl

I have never been to the South, but I imagine this bowl will bring you some of that Southern comfort. The creamy polenta topped with the sweet barbecued cauliflower and savory greens . . . each bite is like a warm hug. The black-eyed peas and pickled red onion round it out, so nothing is missing. You will love this filling bowl!

SERVES 2

QUICK-PICKLED ONIONS

½ cup (80 g) thinly sliced red onion

½ cup (120 ml) water

¼ cup (60 ml) distilled white vinegar

Pinch of salt

POLENTA

4 cups (946 ml) vegetable broth

1 cup (175 g) dried polenta (not instant)

2 tbsp (28 g) vegan butter

Salt and freshly ground black pepper

VEGGIES

1 tbsp (14 g) coconut oil for collards, plus 2 tbsp (30 ml), melted, for cauliflower

1 small yellow onion, diced

Salt and freshly ground black pepper

5 cloves garlic, minced

6 to 7 collard leaves, stemmed and chopped into 2" (5-cm) pieces

1½ cups (355 ml) vegetable broth

1 tsp distilled white vinegar or apple cider vinegar

¼ tsp ground cumin

¼ tsp crushed red pepper flakes

1 large head cauliflower, chopped into florets

⅓ cup (85 g) barbecue sauce, plus more for serving

BEANS

1 (15-oz [425-g]) can black-eyed peas, drained and rinsed

½ tsp ground cumin

½ tsp garlic powder

½ tsp smoked paprika

Salt and freshly ground black pepper

Make the quick-pickled onions: In a small jar or bowl, combine the sliced onion, water, vinegar and salt. Mix well and set aside.

Preheat the oven to 450°F (230°C).

Make the polenta: In a medium-sized soup pot, bring the vegetable broth to a boil, then slowly add the polenta, using a whisk to separate the grains. Once it's all mixed in with no clumps and starting to thicken, about 5 minutes, cover the pot. Lower the heat to a simmer and cook for another 30 minutes, whisking every 5 or 6 minutes. Once it's too thick to whisk, use a wooden spoon instead. When finished cooking, it will have a creamy texture. Stir in the butter and season with salt and black pepper to taste. Set aside.

Make the veggies: In a separate medium-sized soup pot, melt a tablespoon (14 g) of the coconut oil over medium heat. Once hot, add the onion and cook for 3 to 4 minutes. Season with salt and black pepper to taste, then add the garlic, collards, vegetable broth, vinegar, cumin and red pepper flakes. Mix well and bring to a boil, lower the heat to a simmer and cook for 17 to 25 minutes, or until the liquid is almost evaporated and the greens are tender.

Meanwhile, in a bowl, toss the cauliflower with the 2 tablespoons (30 ml) of melted oil and the barbecue sauce. Lay out the florets in a single layer on a baking sheet and roast in the oven for 15 to 20 minutes, or until crispy and caramelized.

Make the beans: In a small bowl, combine the black-eyed peas with the cumin, garlic, smoked paprika and salt and black pepper to taste. Mix well.

Divide the polenta, collards, cauliflower and beans equally between 2 serving bowls. Top with the pickled red onions and drizzle some more barbecue sauce on the cauliflower. Serve immediately.

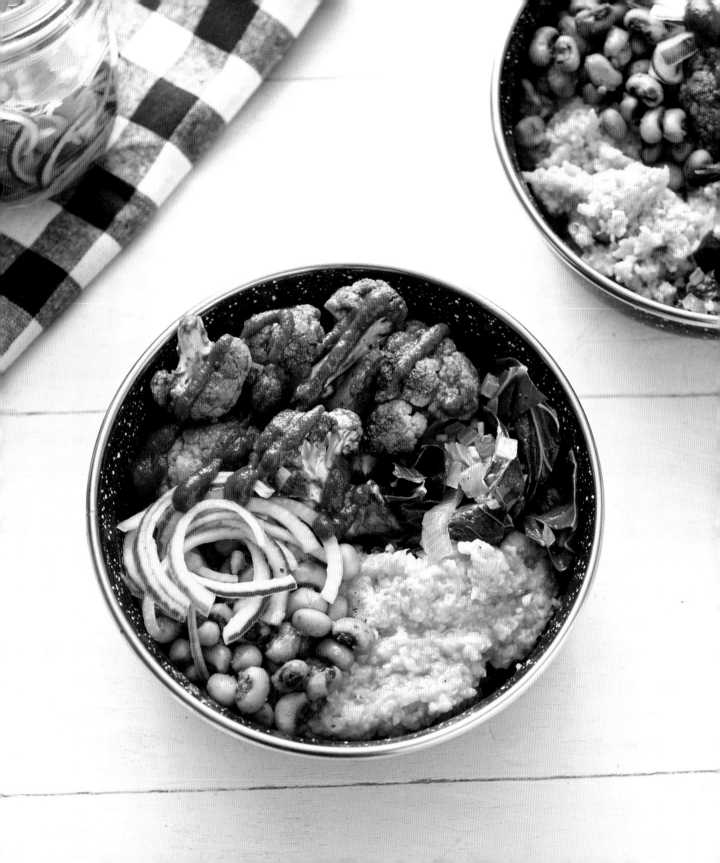

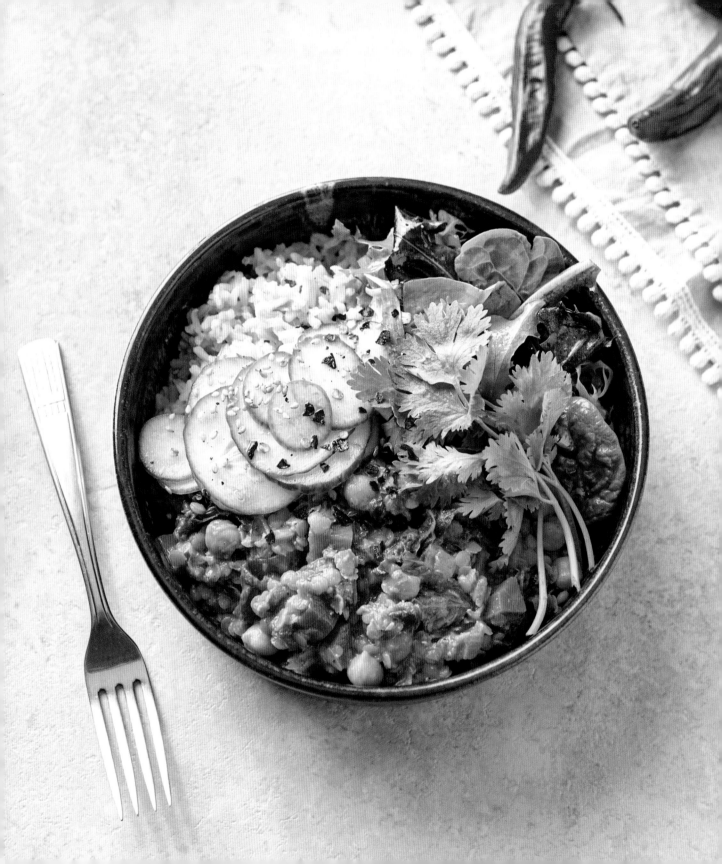

Crowd-Pleasing Curry Bowl

When first coming up with this recipe, I was not consciously trying to combine Indian and east Asian flavors, but that's what happened, and I am not mad about it. There is so much umami flavor from the garbanzo bean and lentil curry, and it is perfectly balanced by the sweet, creamy coconut rice and the crunchy and bright cucumbers. You seriously won't want to stop eating it! Also, if you are not in the mood to make the whole bowl, the curry is absolutely delicious on its own.

SERVES 6

COCONUT RICE

2 cups (380 g) uncooked brown jasmine rice

1 cup (240 ml) vegetable broth

1½ cups (355 ml) water

2 cups (475 ml) coconut cream

Big pinch of salt

GARBANZO BEAN & LENTIL CURRY

2 tbsp (28 g) coconut oil or (30 ml) olive oil

1 large onion, diced

4 to 5 medium-sized carrots, peeled and chopped

Salt

3 to 4 cloves garlic, minced

1½ tsp (3 g) grated (preferred) or minced fresh ginger

2 tbsp (13 g) curry powder (Indian variety with turmeric)

½ tsp crushed red pepper flakes

2 cups (475 ml) vegetable broth

1 (15-oz [425-g]) can coconut cream

1 (28-oz [800-g]) can diced tomatoes

1½ cups (338 g) dried red lentils

1 (15-oz [425-g]) can garbanzo beans

3 cups (201 g) loosely packed chopped kale

Freshly ground black pepper

CUCUMBERS

1 English cucumber, thinly sliced

½ cup (120 ml) rice vinegar

1 tsp sesame seeds

Salt and freshly ground black pepper

MIXED GREENS

6 cups (338 g) mixed greens

2 tbsp (30 ml) rice wine vinegar

2 tbsp (30 ml) toasted sesame oil

GARNISHES

Fresh cilantro

Crushed red pepper flakes

Make the rice: In a medium-sized saucepan, combine the rice, vegetable broth, water, coconut cream and salt. Bring to a boil, then cover and lower the heat to a simmer. Cook until all the liquid is evaporated, 35 to 40 minutes. Set aside.

Make the curry: In a large soup pot, melt the coconut or olive oil over medium heat. Once hot, add the onion and carrots. Cook for 3 to 5 minutes and season generously with salt. Add the garlic, ginger, curry powder and red pepper flakes. Cook, stirring well, for another minute, then add the vegetable broth, coconut cream, diced tomatoes and lentils. Bring to a boil, then cover and lower the heat to a simmer. Cook for 12 to 15 minutes, or until the lentils are cooked through. Add the garbanzo beans and kale and season generously with salt and black pepper. Taste and see whether you want to adjust the flavors.

While the rice and curry cook, make the cucumbers. In a bowl, combine the sliced cucumber with the vinegar, sesame seeds and salt and black pepper to taste and stir well. Set aside.

Then make the mixed greens: Combine the mixed greens in a bowl with the vinegar and sesame oil, and toss well to evenly coat. Set aside.

To build your bowls, divide the rice equally among 6 serving bowls and top with a big scoop of the curry, then the cucumbers and mixed greens. Garnish with cilantro and red pepper flakes and serve.

Spring Roll Bowl

To say that I like spring rolls would be an understatement. I love spring rolls. But making them at home can sometimes be a little too labor intensive for me. My style of at-home cooking is easy and relatively quick. With this bowl, you get all the excitement, fun, flavor and color of a spring roll, without the fuss of rolling them up in rice paper, unless you like that part, of course. The sweet crunchy vegetables with the delicious fresh herbs totally shine when combined with the tangy peanut sauce. Everything is tied together perfectly with the vermicelli rice noodles and it's made a filling meal with the tofu. You'll likely have this on high rotation!

───────── SERVES 4 ─────────

PEANUT SAUCE

½ cup (130 g) creamy peanut butter

¼ cup (60 ml) water

2 tbsp (30 ml) tamari or soy sauce

2 tbsp (30 ml) pure maple syrup

2 tbsp (30 ml) lime juice

1 tsp garlic powder

TOFU

1 (15.5-oz [439-g]) package extra-firm tofu

¼ cup (55 g) coconut oil

¼ cup (60 ml) tamari or soy sauce

½ tsp garlic powder

NOODLES

8 oz (225 g) dried vermicelli rice noodles

BOWLS

1 medium-sized green cabbage, thinly sliced

1 cup (40 g) loosely packed chopped fresh mint

¾ cup (30 g) loosely packed chopped fresh basil

½ cup (20 g) loosely packed chopped fresh cilantro

3 medium-sized carrots, peeled and shredded

2 small radishes, thinly sliced

1 medium-sized red bell pepper, seeded and julienned

1 English cucumber, julienned

1 jalapeño pepper, seeded and diced

GARNISHES

Green onion

Sriracha

Fresh cilantro

Crushed peanuts

Make the sauce: In a small bowl, vigorously whisk together the peanut butter, water, tamari, maple syrup, lime juice and garlic powder until well combined. If the peanut butter is not at room temperature, warm it in the microwave so it's easy to blend.

Make the tofu: Remove the tofu from the packaging and drain the water. Then wrap the tofu block in a clean towel or several paper towels. Press down to remove as much liquid as possible, and then cut into 1-inch (2.5-cm) cubes. In a large skillet, melt the coconut oil over medium-high heat. Once hot, add the cubed tofu. Let cook for 5 minutes, then toss or flip to another side. Cook for another 5 minutes and then toss or flip once more. Cook for another 3 minutes. Add the tamari and garlic powder and stir well. Remove from the heat and set aside.

Make the noodles: Bring a medium-sized saucepan of salted water to a boil. Add the rice noodles and cook according to the package instructions, then drain and run some cold water over them to stop the cooking. Set aside.

Make the bowls: In a large bowl, combine the cabbage, mint, basil and cilantro. Toss to mix well, then divide among 4 serving bowls. Divide the noodles and tofu equally among the bowls and top each bowl with the carrots, radishes, bell pepper, cucumber and jalapeño. Add the sauce on top and garnish with green onion, sriracha, cilantro and crushed peanuts. Serve immediately.

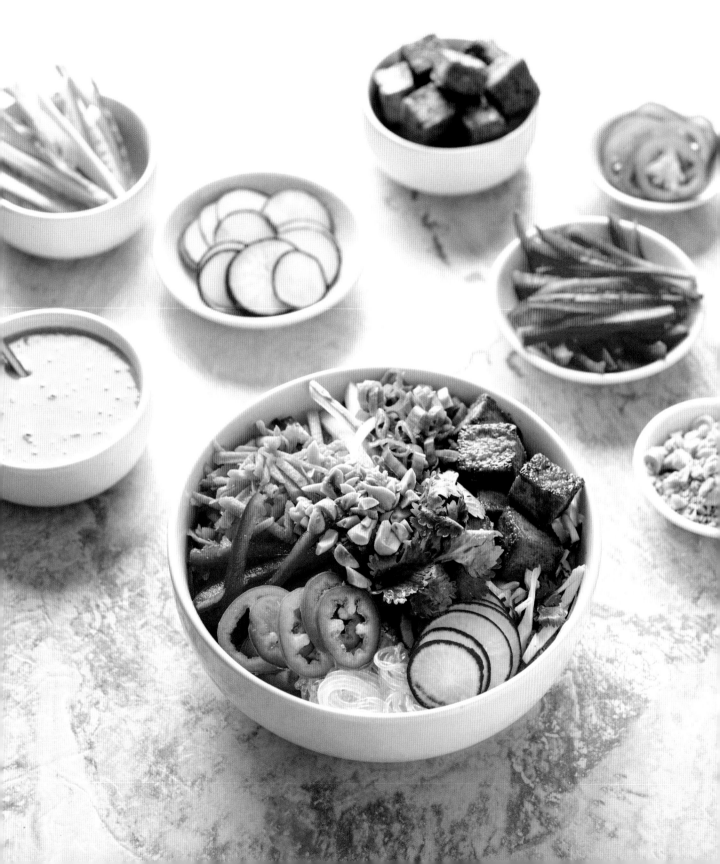

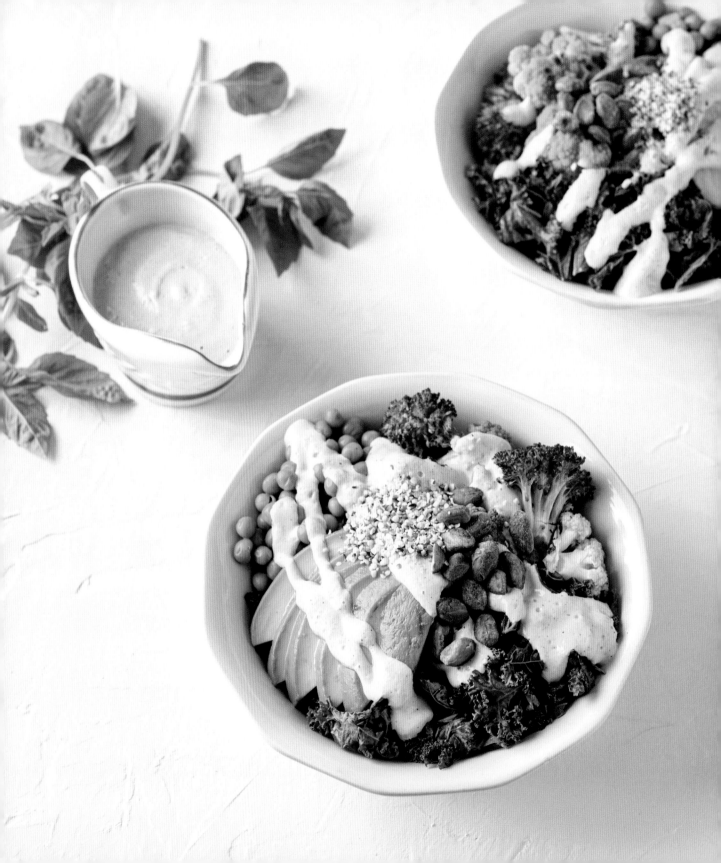

The Green Machine

For the longest time, I struggled to truly enjoy eating nutrient-dense foods because I was always motivated from a place of shame about my body and the idea that I needed to lose weight. It wasn't until I was motivated from an authentic place of wanting to honor myself that it all shifted. Now, a bowl loaded to the brim with green veggies excites me. And this one is a real winner! The savory yet sweet basil tahini sauce beautifully coats each vegetable, enhancing the already amazing flavor. The creamy avocado is balanced out by all the crunch, which makes this a texture powerhouse—something not to be overlooked when it comes to food. And since this is so easy to make, I would slide it into the category of lazy-fancy, and perfect to impress some hungry dinner guests.

SERVES 4

BASIL-TAHINI SAUCE

⅓ cup (80 g) tahini

1 cup (21 g) tightly packed chopped fresh basil leaves

2 cloves garlic

½ cup (120 ml) avocado oil

3 tbsp (45 ml) apple cider vinegar

1 tbsp (15 ml) pure maple syrup

1 tsp curry powder (Indian variety with turmeric)

½ tsp smoked paprika

Pinch of cayenne

½ cup (120 ml) water

Salt and freshly ground black pepper

VEGGIES

6 cups (402 g) broccoli florets

1 head green or Romanesco cauliflower, chopped into florets

¼ cup (60 ml) melted coconut oil, divided

Salt and freshly ground black pepper

10 cups (670 g) loosely packed chopped kale leaves

1½ cups (225 g) sweet peas

1 ripe avocado, peeled, pitted and sliced

GARNISHES

Hemp seeds

Pistachios

Preheat the oven to 450°F (230°C).

Make the sauce: In a blender, combine the tahini, basil, garlic, avocado oil, vinegar, maple syrup, curry powder, smoked paprika, cayenne and water. Blend until well combined. Season with salt and pepper to taste.

Lay out the broccoli and green cauliflower florets in a single layer on a baking sheet. Top with 2 tablespoons (30 ml) of the coconut oil. Toss to coat, season with salt and pepper to taste, then roast in the oven for 12 to 18 minutes, or until fork-tender and crispy and browned on one side. Set aside.

In a large skillet, melt the remaining 2 tablespoons (30 ml) of coconut oil over medium heat. Add the kale and cook for 7 to 9 minutes, or until the leaves are wilted; season with salt and pepper to taste, then set aside.

Divide the broccoli, green cauliflower, kale, peas and avocado equally between 4 serving bowls, then drizzle with the sauce. Garnish with hemp seeds and pistachios. Serve immediately.

Harissa Curry Bowl

This is one of those recipes that came together on a whim. We had loads of fresh produce in the house at the time, but I wasn't exactly sure how I would cook them all. After digging around in the cabinet, I found some coconut cream and harissa and knew immediately it was a match made in flavor heaven. The sweetness of the coconut marries together perfectly with the spicy harissa, and results in a delicious take on classic red Thai curry. The mushrooms, kale and garbanzo bean provide great texture and nutrients, while the quinoa makes it a filling and well-rounded dish. This is so perfect for an easy weeknight meal.

— SERVES 2 —

QUINOA

1½ cups (260 g) uncooked quinoa

3 cups (710 ml) vegetable broth

2 tsp (4 g) curry powder

2 tsp (6 g) garlic powder

Salt and freshly ground black pepper

HARISSA CURRY

1 tbsp (14 g) coconut oil

¾ cup (120 g) diced white onion

Salt and freshly ground black pepper

4 cloves garlic, minced

3 cups (210 g) sliced cremini mushrooms

3 cups (208 g) tightly packed chopped kale leaves

1 to 2 tbsp (15 to 30 g) harissa paste

1 (13.5-oz [400-ml]) can coconut cream

1½ cups (355 ml) vegetable broth

1 tsp pure maple syrup

1 tsp garlic powder

1 (15-oz [425-g]) can garbanzo beans

Salt and freshly ground black pepper

GARNISH

Green onion

Make the quinoa: In a medium-sized saucepan, combine the quinoa and vegetable broth and bring to a boil. Cover, lower the heat to simmer and cook until all the liquid is evaporated, 10 to 15 minutes. Then, add the curry powder, garlic powder, salt and pepper to taste, mix well and set aside.

Meanwhile, make the harissa curry: In a separate medium-sized saucepan, melt the coconut oil over medium heat. Once hot, add the onion and cook for 3 to 5 minutes. Season with a pinch of salt and pepper, then add the garlic and cook for another 30 seconds.

Add the mushrooms and cook, stirring occasionally, for 5 to 7 minutes, or until their liquid starts to release. Add the kale leaves and cook, stirring frequently, until they are cooked down, 6 to 8 minutes.

Add the harissa, coconut cream, vegetable broth, maple syrup and garlic powder and stir well to combine. Bring to a boil, then lower the heat to a simmer and cook for 5 minutes. Add the garbanzo beans and season to taste with salt and pepper, adjusting any of the seasonings if desired.

Divide the quinoa and vegetable curry mixture between 2 serving bowls and top with green onion.

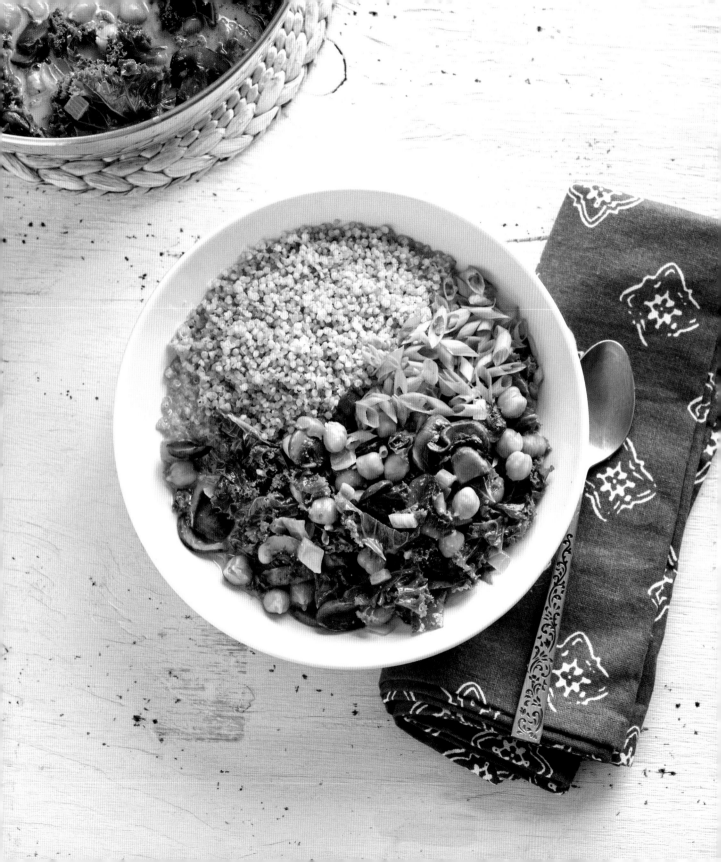

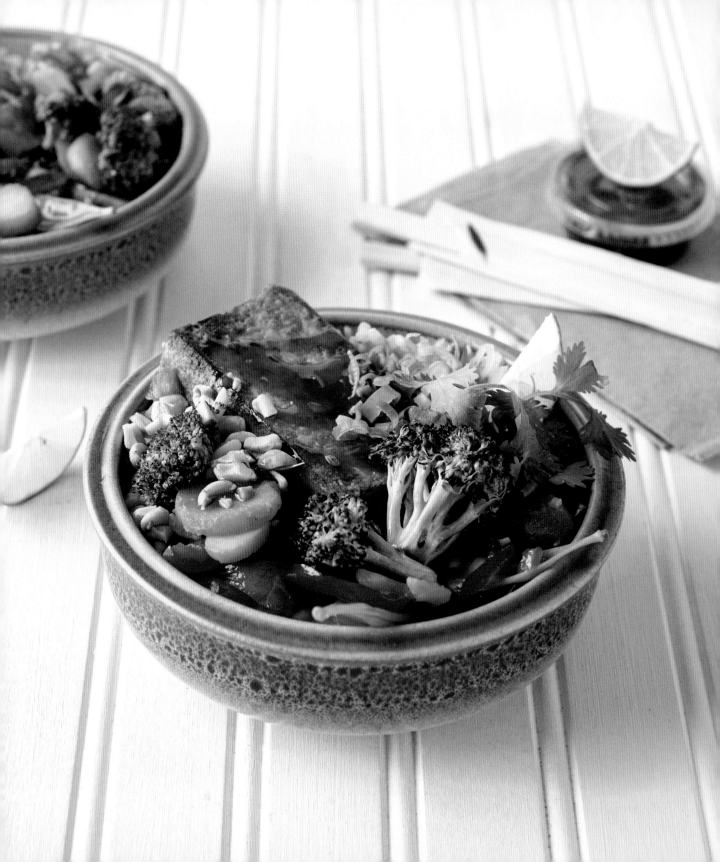

Tangy Tofu Bowl

I'll be honest, there isn't great Chinese take-out in the part of Los Angeles where I live, so whenever I am in the mood for some, this is my go-to. The cooking method for the tofu leaves it with the perfect texture—soft inside, crispy outside—that pairs perfectly with the sauce and the crunchy veggies. And we have the usual suspects like broccoli, red bell pepper, snow peas and water chestnuts—an absolute must, even if it means a separate trip to the Asian market. Serve it on a bed of rice and you're left with a better-than-delivery, take-out-style meal!

SERVES 4

TOFU & TANGY SESAME SAUCE

1 (15.5-oz [439-g]) package extra-firm tofu (organic and sprouted preferred)

⅓ cup (80 ml) tamari or soy sauce

⅓ cup (80 ml) toasted sesame oil

⅓ cup (80 ml) apple cider vinegar

1 tbsp (15 ml) pure maple syrup

Juice of 1 lime

Pinch of red pepper flakes

Salt and freshly ground black pepper

3 tbsp (42 g) coconut oil

VEGGIES

2 tbsp (28 g) coconut oil

½ cup (80 g) diced onion

Salt and freshly ground black pepper

4 cloves garlic, minced

1 tsp minced fresh ginger

3 cups (213 g) broccoli florets

1 medium-sized red bell pepper, seeded and thinly sliced

1½ cups (240 g) snow peas

2 (8-oz [225-g]) cans sliced water chestnuts, drained and rinsed

¼ cup (60 ml) tamari or soy sauce

TO SERVE & GARNISHES

4 cups (780 g) cooked short-grain brown rice, for serving

Sweet chili sauce, or hot sauce of choice

Green onion

Fresh cilantro

Lime wedges

Chopped cashews

Preheat the oven to 450°F (230°C).

Press the tofu: Drain the water from the tofu, then wrap it in a clean dish towel or paper towel. Place a book or two on top to help squeeze out the moisture from the tofu. Let it sit for 5 minutes, swapping out the towel for new dry ones, if necessary.

While the tofu is being pressed, make the sauce: In a small bowl, vigorously whisk together the tamari, sesame oil, vinegar, maple syrup, lime juice, red pepper flakes and salt and black pepper to taste, until well combined, 1 to 2 minutes. Set aside.

Slice the tofu into ¾-inch (2-cm) rectangular "steaks." Pat dry with a clean towel, if necessary. In a cast-iron skillet, melt the coconut oil over medium-high heat. You want there to be enough oil to coat the bottom and prevent the tofu from sticking, so do not be shy here. Once hot, gently transfer the tofu steaks to the skillet and let fry and sizzle for 6 minutes. Then, using a thin spatula, gently flip each steak and fry for another 6 minutes on the opposite side.

Remove from the heat and pour ⅓ cup (80 ml) of the tangy sauce on top, reserving the rest of the sauce for the veggies. Transfer the skillet to the oven and bake for 10 to 12 minutes, or until crispy and golden brown.

Meanwhile, make the veggies: In a large skillet or wok, melt the coconut oil over medium heat. Once hot, add the onion and cook for 3 to 5 minutes, or until translucent and fragrant. Season with salt and pepper to taste. Add the garlic and ginger, and stir-fry for 30 to 60 seconds. Add the broccoli and bell pepper and cook for 6 to 8 minutes, stirring occasionally. Add the snow peas and cook for another 5 to 7 minutes. Add the water chestnuts and the tamari and mix well. Cook for another 2 to 3 minutes, then add the remaining sauce and toss to evenly coat the veggies. Taste and see whether you want to adjust the seasonings or add any salt and pepper.

Remove from the heat. Divide the rice, veggies and tofu equally among 4 bowls, add chili sauce, green onion, cilantro, lime wedges and cashews as desired and serve.

Jicama Nacho Bowl

Sometimes, I think jicama was created just for the sole purpose of being used as chips in nacho recipes. I love to slice raw jicama thinly with a mandoline—it's so crispy, light and refreshing, it makes the perfect vehicle for all the toppings. The cashew sour cream and nacho cheese pair perfectly with the flavorful walnut taco meat; even carnivores will enjoy this. Add the usual toppings, such as salsa and guacamole, and you have yourself an interesting and fun take on traditional nachos!

--- SERVES 2 ---

CASHEW SOUR CREAM & NACHO CHEESE

1 cup (140 g) raw cashews, soaked in very hot water for 12 minutes (see Note)

⅓ cup plus 2 tbsp (110 ml) water

Juice of 1 lemon

2 cloves garlic

1 tbsp (8 g) nutritional yeast

1 tsp apple cider vinegar

Salt and freshly ground black pepper

1 tbsp (15 ml) hot sauce of choice

WALNUT TACO MEAT

1 cup (55 g) dried sun-dried tomatoes (not oil-packed), soaked in hot water for 5 minutes

1½ cups (150 g) raw walnuts

½ jalapeño pepper, seeded and diced

1 tbsp (9 g) garlic powder

1 tbsp (7 g) ground cumin

1 tsp smoked paprika

¼ tsp cayenne pepper

Salt and freshly ground black pepper

NACHOS

1 large jicama, peeled and sliced very thinly with a mandoline (preferred) or knife

1 cup (260 g) prepared salsa

1 cup (225 g) prepared guacamole, or 1 ripe avocado, peeled, pitted and diced

½ cup (80 g) diced red onion

½ jalapeño pepper, seeded if preferred, and diced

GARNISHES

Fresh cilantro

Green onion

Lime wedges

Make the sour cream and nacho cheese: Rinse and drain the soaked cashews. In a high-speed blender, combine the cashews, fresh water, lemon juice, garlic and nutritional yeast. Blend on high speed until smooth. Divide the mixture equally between 2 bowls. To one bowl, add the vinegar plus salt and pepper to taste and mix well; this is your sour cream. To the other bowl, add the hot sauce, salt and pepper to taste and mix well; this is your nacho cheese. Set both aside.

Make the taco meat: While the sun-dried tomatoes soak, place the walnuts in a food processor fitted with the S blade and pulse in 5-second bursts, 5 times, or until the walnuts look like a crumble mixture but not a flour. Transfer to a bowl and set aside.

Drain all but ¼ cup (60 ml) of the water from the sun-dried tomatoes. Place the drained sun-dried tomatoes and their reserved soaking water, jalapeño, garlic, cumin, smoked paprika, cayenne and salt and black pepper in the food processor. Process on high speed for 30 seconds to 1 minute, or until a paste forms, stopping to scrape down the sides, if necessary. Transfer the mixture to the bowl of walnuts and mix well.

Build your nachos: In each of the 2 serving bowls, lay out a single layer of jicama. Drizzle with some of the sour cream and nacho cheese and a little of the walnut taco meat. Repeat another 2 or 3 times, until all the jicama is used, making sure there is some sour cream, nacho cheese and walnut taco meat left to put on top of each stack of nachos. Then, top each plate with salsa and guacamole and garnish with diced red onion, jalapeño, cilantro, green onion and lime wedges. Serve immediately.

Note: If you do not have a high-speed blender, soak your cashews for an hour or overnight, to protect your blender.

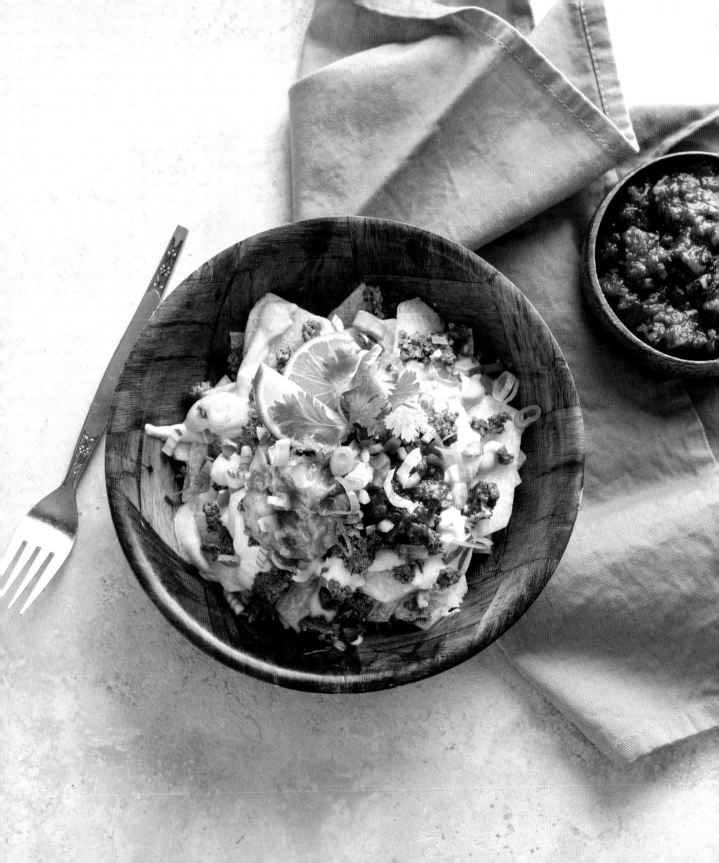

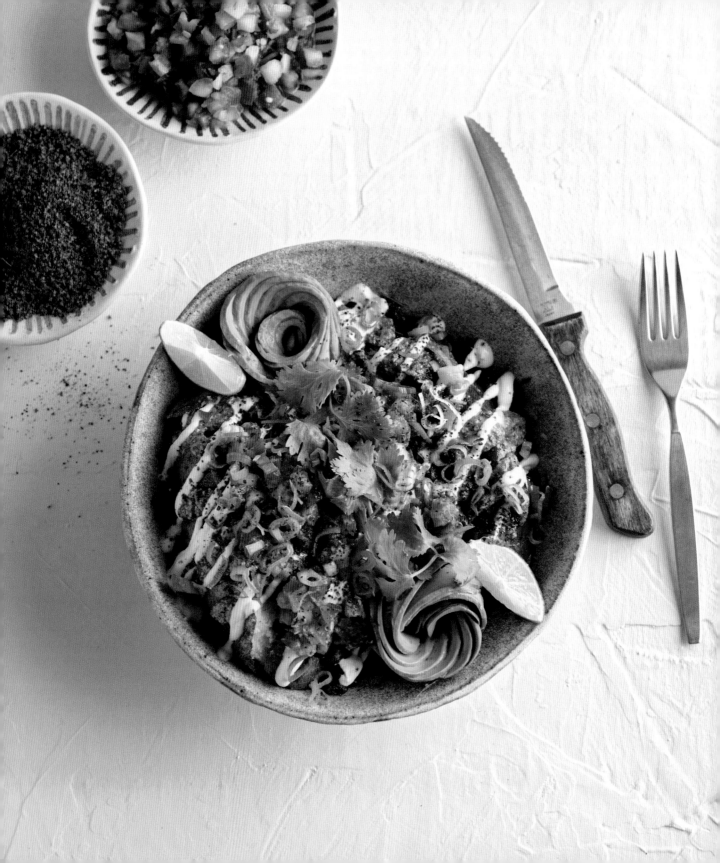

Loaded Baked Potato Bowl

I am a huge fan of potatoes! They are affordable, delicious and one of the very first carb-heavy whole foods I allowed myself to eat without guilt—which was a huge deal for me back in the day when I was just entering recovery. This bowl is paying homage to the humble spud and simple cooking method of baked potatoes. There are two delicious sauces: a rich and vibrant cashew sour cream and a spicy and bright cilantro pesto (mix them together for a seriously good combo). It's made a balanced bowl by adding black beans and avocado. Garnished with just the right toppings—lime, green onion, cilantro and Tajín—to tie all the flavors together!

SERVES 2

POTATOES

2 large russet potatoes

2 large sweet potatoes

2 tbsp (28 g) vegan butter

Salt

CASHEW SOUR CREAM

1 recipe Cashew Sour Cream & Nacho Cheese (page 42)

1 tsp apple cider vinegar

SPICY CILANTRO PESTO

¼ cup (34 g) raw pine nuts

2 cloves garlic

1 tbsp (8 g) nutritional yeast

1 tbsp (4 g) crushed red pepper flakes

¼ tsp cayenne pepper

3 cups (120 g) loosely packed fresh cilantro

2 tbsp (30 ml) fresh lime juice

⅓ cup (80 ml) olive oil

Salt and freshly ground black pepper

BOWL

1 (15-oz [425 g]) can black beans, drained and rinsed

½ tsp ground cumin

½ tsp garlic powder

½ tsp smoked paprika

Salt and freshly ground black pepper

TO SERVE AND GARNISHES

1 ripe avocado, peeled, pitted and thinly sliced, for serving

Pico de gallo salsa

Green onion

Fresh cilantro

Lime wedges

Chile lime or Tajín seasoning

Bake the potatoes: Preheat the oven to 425°F (220°C). Using a fork, pierce each potato 2 or 3 times, then rub each one with some butter and salt. Place on a baking sheet and bake for about 45 minutes, or until fork-tender and cooked through. The sweet potatoes will cook more quickly, so check them at around the 30- to 35-minute mark. When each potato is cooked, remove from the oven and set aside.

While the potatoes bake, make the sour cream: Follow the directions on page 42 as written, except do not divide the cashew cream in half or add the hot sauce. Simply add the additional teaspoon of apple cider vinegar. Set in the fridge to chill while prepping everything else.

Make the spicy cilantro pesto: In a food processor fitted with an S blade, combine the pine nuts, garlic, nutritional yeast, red pepper flakes and cayenne and pulse in 10-second bursts, 3 times. Add the cilantro and lime juice and pulse in 6-second bursts, 4 times. With the food processor on low speed, slowly pour the oil through the center of the lid and mix until well combined. Season with salt and black pepper to taste. Set aside.

Make the beans: Place the black beans in a microwave-safe bowl and microwave for 1 to 2 minutes. Add the cumin, garlic powder and smoked paprika, stir well and season with salt and black pepper to taste.

Once the baked potatoes are done, slice them almost all the way in half and use a fork to mash some of the flesh of each. Divide between 2 serving bowls. Layer the beans and then the sour cream and cilantro pesto equally in each bowl, then top each with half of a sliced avocado. Garnish with salsa, green onion, cilantro, lime wedges and chili lime seasoning.

Farro Fattoush Bowl

I was once told that there is no such thing as too much sumac! And after making this recipe, you will likely understand what I mean. It is the tiny but big star that brings so much flavor to this grain bowl and is a staple in Middle Eastern cooking. It has a tart, lemony taste that is the perfect pairing with the fresh tomatoes and crunchy cucumber and radish. The herbaceous parsley and onion paired with the sweet mint adds a lovely complexity. It's balanced out with the farro, which takes the place of pita chips in a more traditional fattoush-style salad and transforms it into a grain bowl. This is a perfect make-ahead recipe for lunch or a potluck. If you can't find sumac at your local market, you can get it in Middle Eastern stores or at online retailers. It's worth the extra effort!

SERVES 4

SUMAC VINAIGRETTE

¼ cup (60 ml) fresh lemon juice

2 tsp (5 g) ground sumac

½ tsp ground cinnamon

½ tsp garlic powder

½ tsp maple syrup

¾ cup (180 ml) extra virgin olive oil

Salt and freshly ground black pepper

BOWL

2 cups (400 g) uncooked farro

1 English cucumber, cut into bite-size pieces

3 radishes, thinly sliced and cut into bite-size pieces

3 Roma tomatoes, cut into bite-size pieces

⅓ cup (55 g) thinly sliced red onion

1 cup (60 g) chopped fresh parsley leaves

1 cup (40 g) chopped fresh mint leaves

3 green onions, thinly sliced

½ tsp ground sumac

Salt and freshly ground black pepper

4 cups (220 g) chopped romaine lettuce

GARNISHES

Lemon wedges

White sesame seeds

Ground sumac

Crushed pistachios or almonds

Make the sumac vinaigrette: In a small bowl, combine the lemon juice, sumac, cinnamon, garlic powder and maple syrup. Slowly whisk in the olive oil until well incorporated. Season with salt and pepper to taste. Set aside.

Make the bowl: Bring a large pot of salted water to a boil, add the farro, cover and lower the heat to a simmer. Cook for 25 to 30 minutes, or until tender and cooked through. Remove from the heat, rinse with cold water and transfer to a large bowl.

Add the cucumber, radishes, tomatoes, red onion, parsley, mint, green onions, sumac and salt and pepper to taste, to the farro. Add three-quarters of the vinaigrette and mix well.

Divide the chopped romaine equally among 4 serving bowls and add one-quarter of the remaining vinaigrette on each bed of lettuce. Divide the farro mixture among the bowls and garnish with a lemon wedge, white sesame seeds, ground sumac and pistachios.

If making ahead of time, mix everything as directed, but store the dressing separately until ready to serve. Everything will keep well in airtight containers in the fridge for 5 to 7 days.

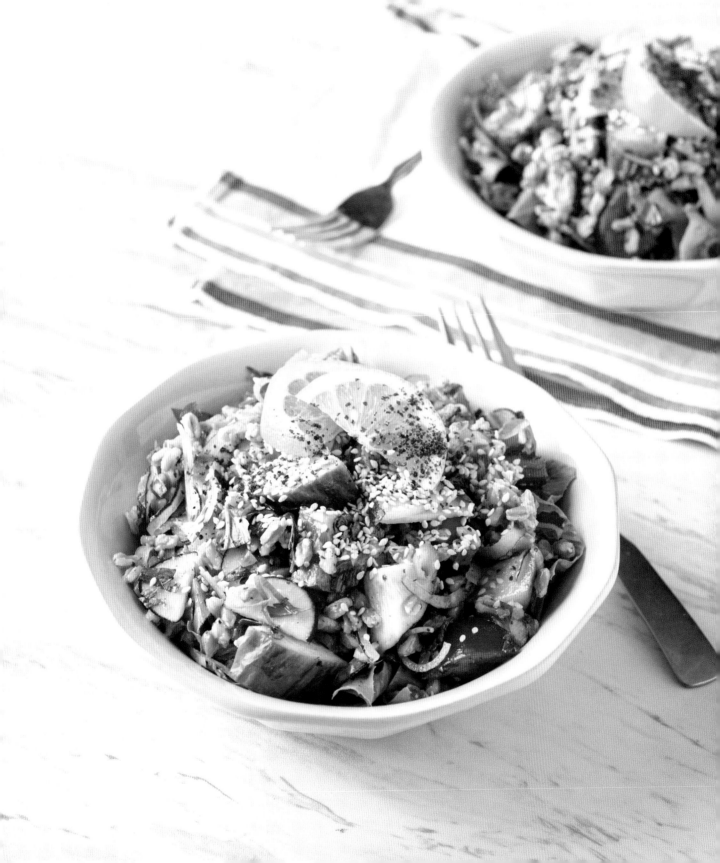

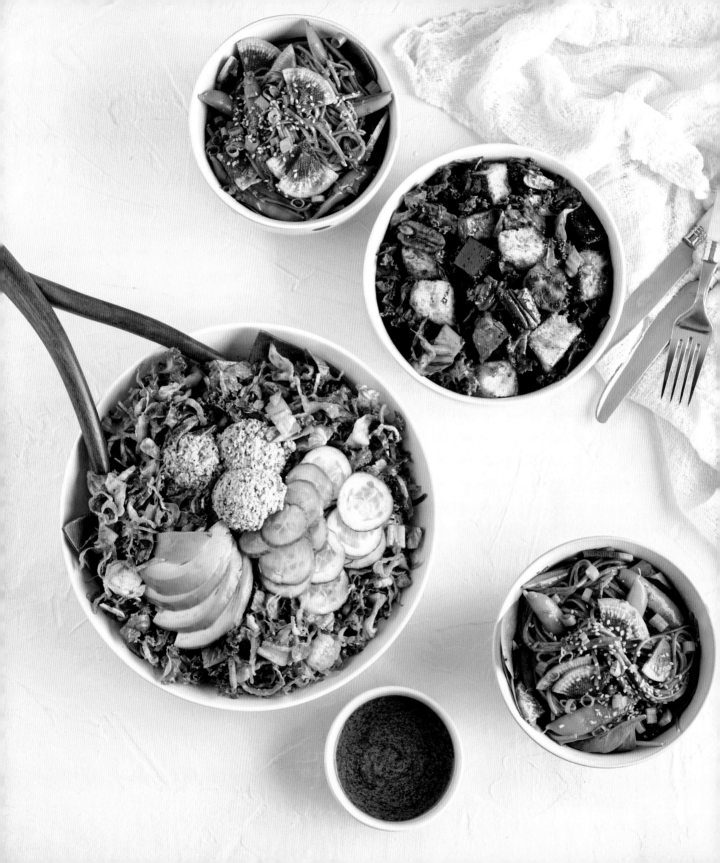

Vibrant, Nourishing Salad Bowls

Many people think that salads are boring, and I get it, because sometimes they are! But, rest assured these salads are anything but and they just might become loved by some of your non-salad-loving friends. I know my boyfriend was pleasantly surprised by how much he enjoyed these and even more surprised by his own request for me to make them again!

Each is fused together with a variety of ingredients offering up unexpected flavor combinations, such as my Spring Vegetable Panzanella (page 58), or taking a fun spin on a tried-and-true classic, such as my Goddess Greens (page 50). Whichever you choose (or should you make them all), may I suggest that you eat your salad from a big beautiful bowl for ultimate satisfaction. I find that eating from a plate just isn't the same!

Goddess Greens

This is my spin on the trendy green goddess salad and it truly is fit for a goddess. The bright and zingy cilantro vinaigrette not only pops next to the creamy avocado, it also balances out the bitterness of the greens, tying everything together. And just to keep it interesting and bursting with brain health benefits from the walnuts, there is the herb pâté on top. You will happily be swimming in this sea of green!

── **SERVES 4** ──

HERB PÂTÉ

2 cups (250 g) raw walnuts, soaked in very hot water for 10 minutes

⅓ cup (80 ml) water

2 cloves garlic

¼ cup (60 ml) fresh lemon juice

2 tbsp (30 ml) olive oil

Pinch of red pepper flakes

1½ cups (60 g) fresh cilantro

12 big fresh basil leaves

2 green onions

Salt

CILANTRO VINAIGRETTE

2 shallots, roughly chopped

4 cups (164 g) tightly packed fresh cilantro leaves

1 green onion

2 cloves garlic

1 tsp red pepper flakes

1 cup (240 ml) avocado oil or grapeseed oil

⅓ cup (80 ml) red wine vinegar

Salt and freshly ground black pepper

SALAD

4 cups (275 g) tightly packed shredded kale

4 cups (360 g) tightly packed shredded Brussels sprouts

8 cups (440 g) chopped romaine lettuce

2 ripe avocados, sliced

1 English cucumber, thinly sliced

Make the herb pâté: Rinse and drain the walnuts. Place the walnuts in a food processor and grind in 10-second bursts, 2 times, until they are reduced to big crumbs. Add the fresh water, garlic, lemon juice, olive oil, red pepper flakes, cilantro, basil, green onions and salt to taste. Pulse, stopping to scrape down the sides if necessary, in 10-second bursts, 3 times, or until slightly smooth but still a little chunky and resembling canned tuna. Set aside.

Make the vinaigrette: In a high-speed blender, combine the shallots, cilantro, green onion, garlic, red pepper flakes, avocado oil and vinegar. Blend at high speed until smooth. Add salt and black pepper to taste. Set aside.

Make the salad: In a large bowl, mix together the kale, Brussels sprouts and romaine. Add the dressing and toss well. Use tongs, or your hands, to massage the greens with the dressing to soften. Divide the greens equally among 4 serving bowls, top each bowl with half of an avocado and one-quarter of the pâté and divide the cucumber slices among the bowls.

If making ahead of time, mix everything as written, except the avocado, which should be added just before serving. Store the dressing and pâté separately until ready to eat. Everything will keep well in airtight containers in the fridge for 5 to 7 days.

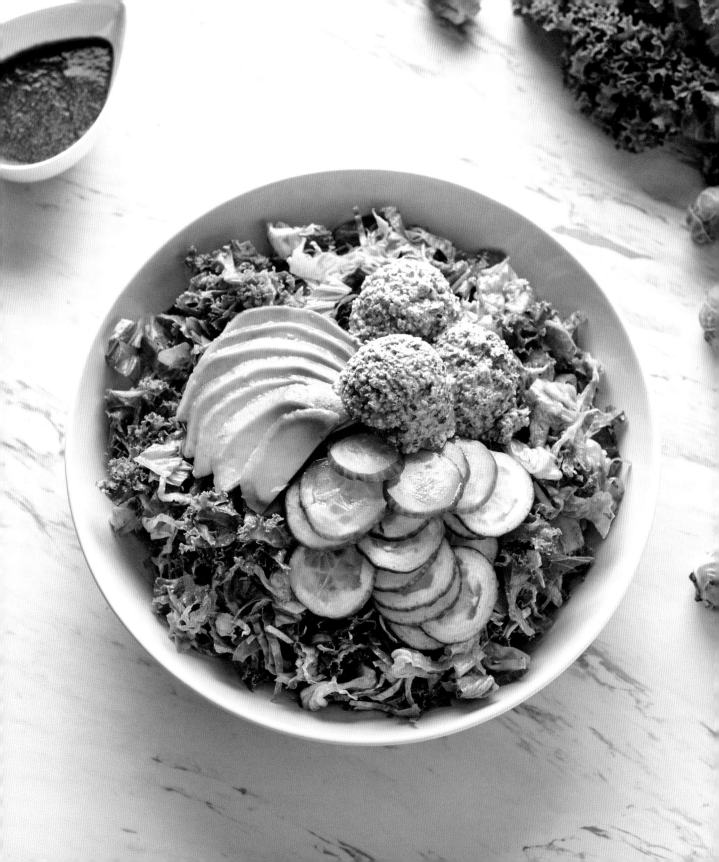

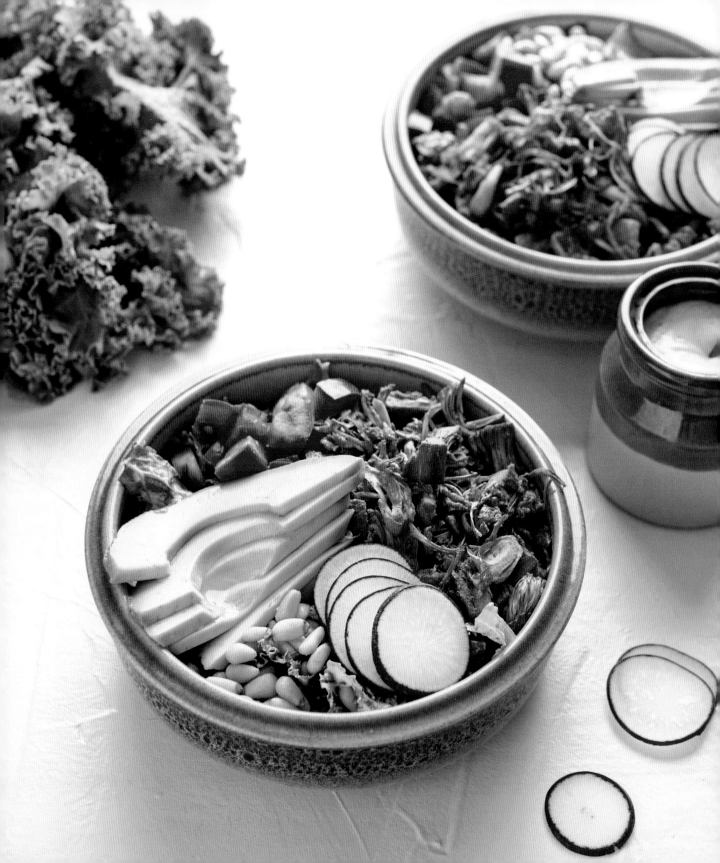

Jackfruit Chicken Kale Caesar

This is easily one of my all-time favorite salads. The cashew Caesar dressing is so good, I could just eat it with a spoon. The classic salad is a star in its own right, but the jackfruit makes this extra special. One of my favorite things is that it is one of the few leafy green salads that is even better the next day!

SERVES 4

JACKFRUIT CHICKEN

2 tbsp (30 ml) melted coconut oil

¾ cup (115 g) diced white onion

1 (20-oz [567-g]) can jackfruit in brine (not syrup), drained and rinsed

3 cloves garlic, grated or minced

½ tsp garlic powder

½ tsp ground cumin

½ tsp smoked paprika

¼ tsp onion powder

⅛ tsp cayenne pepper

2 cups (475 ml) vegetable broth

1 tsp liquid smoke

1 tbsp (15 ml) soy sauce or tamari

Salt and freshly ground black pepper

DRESSING

1 cup (140 g) raw cashews, soaked in very hot water for 12 minutes (see Note)

⅓ cup (80 ml) water, plus more if needed

2 cloves garlic

1 tbsp (8 g) nutritional yeast

1 tsp Worcestershire sauce

1 tsp prepared yellow mustard

1 tsp garlic powder

¼ cup (60 ml) fresh lemon juice

1 tsp freshly ground black pepper

Salt

SALAD

5 cups (335 g) chopped kale

4 cups (220 g) chopped romaine lettuce

1 beefsteak tomato, seeded and diced

1 fresh avocado, peeled, pitted and sliced

½ cup (58 g) thinly sliced radish

⅓ cup (45 g) pine nuts or (48 g) sunflower seeds

Make the jackfruit chicken: In a large, lidded skillet, heat the coconut oil over medium heat. Once hot, add the onion and cook for 4 to 5 minutes. Add the jackfruit, grated garlic, garlic powder, cumin, smoked paprika, onion powder and cayenne and stir well to coat. Cook, uncovered, for 3 to 4 minutes, then add the vegetable broth, liquid smoke and soy sauce. Bring to a boil, cover and lower the heat to a medium simmer over medium-low heat. Cook for 7 minutes and then, using the back of a wooden spoon, start to break up the jackfruit into smaller pieces. If it is still a little tough, cook for another 5 to 6 minutes and break it up again. You want it to be slightly shredded and have some small bite-sized pieces. Once the jackfruit is broken up, simmer, covered, stirring occasionally, until all the liquid has evaporated, about 25 minutes.

About halfway through cooking the jackfruit, preheat the oven to 425°F (220°C) and lightly oil a baking sheet with coconut oil. Once the jackfruit is cooked, lay it out in a single layer on the prepared baking sheet, Season with salt and black pepper to taste and bake for 10 to 15 minutes, stirring halfway through.

Make the dressing: Drain and rinse the cashews. In a high-speed blender, combine the cashews, the fresh water, garlic, nutritional yeast, Worcestershire sauce, mustard, garlic powder, lemon juice, black pepper and salt. Blend on high speed until smooth and creamy.

Make the salad: Place the chopped kale in a large bowl and add the dressing. Using tongs, massage the dressing into the kale, then add the chopped romaine and mix well. Divide equally among 4 serving bowls, then top each bowl with the tomato, jackfruit chicken, avocado, radish and pine nuts. Serve immediately.

Although this does get better a day after adding the dressing, it starts to get soggy by day 3. Keep the dressing separate if you're making this salad for meal prep. Everything keeps well in an airtight container in the fridge for up to a week.

Note: *If you do not have a high-speed blender, soak your cashews for an hour or overnight to protect your blender.*

Energizing Sweet Potato & Greens Salad

Although this salad is good for lunch and dinner, it's one that I frequently make for breakfast! Believe it or not, I wake up in the mood for greens pretty often, so I just go with it. The coconut bacon is so good and makes this extra special plus a little over the top—which, in this case, is a good thing! The lemon tahini is perfect with the sweet potatoes, avocados and mixed greens. This would be a great addition to a beautiful brunch with friends.

SERVES 4

COCONUT BACON

2 cups (170 g) large unsweetened coconut flakes

1 tbsp (15 ml) avocado oil

2 tbsp (30 ml) coconut aminos (preferred), tamari or soy sauce

1 tsp smoked paprika

½ tsp garlic powder

¼ tsp ground cumin

1 tbsp (15 ml) pure maple syrup

½ tsp liquid smoke

Salt and freshly ground black pepper

LEMON TAHINI

⅓ cup (80 ml) avocado or grapeseed oil

¼ cup (60 g) tahini

2 tbsp (30 ml) fresh lemon juice

½ tsp garlic powder

½ tsp Dijon mustard

1 tsp maple syrup

Salt and black pepper to taste

SALAD

8 cups (450 g) tightly packed mixed salad greens

3 cups (400 g) roasted and cubed sweet potato (½" [1.2-cm] cubes)

2 ripe avocados, peeled, pitted and sliced

GARNISHES

Fresh cilantro

Green onion

Make the coconut bacon. Preheat the oven to 325°F (165°C) and line a baking sheet with parchment paper. Combine the coconut flakes, oil, coconut aminos, paprika, garlic powder, ground cumin, maple syrup, liquid smoke, salt and pepper on the prepared baking sheet and toss to evenly coat. Bake for 5 to 6 minutes, then stir and return the pan to the oven. Bake for another 5 to 7 minutes, or until the coconut flakes are crispy and golden brown. Keep an eye on the mixture so it doesn't burn. Remove from the oven and let cool for 10 minutes to crisp up in the air.

Meanwhile, make the dressing: In a small bowl, vigorously whisk together the avocado oil, tahini, lemon juice, garlic powder, Dijon mustard, maple syrup, salt and pepper until well combined.

Make the salad: In a large bowl, combine the salad greens, roasted sweet potato, half of the coconut bacon and half the dressing. Toss well, then divide equally among 4 serving bowls. Evenly divide the remaining coconut bacon, avocado slices and remaining dressing on top of the bowls. Garnish with cilantro and green onion and serve.

If making ahead of time, mix everything as directed, except the avocado, which should be reserved until ready to serve. Store the dressing and the coconut bacon separately. Store the coconut bacon at room temperature on the counter for 5 to 7 days. Everything else will keep well in airtight containers in the fridge for 5 to 7 days.

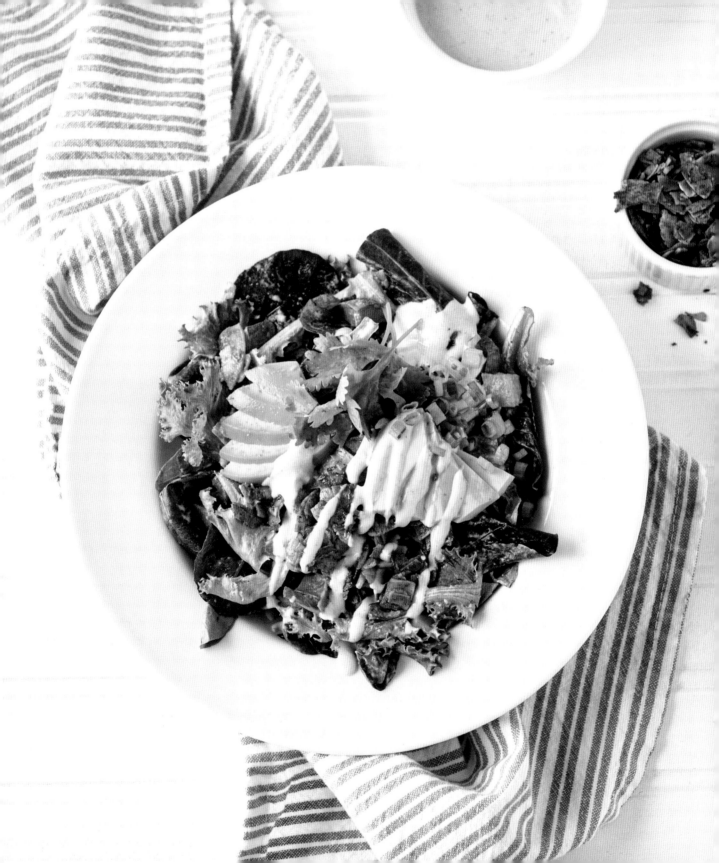

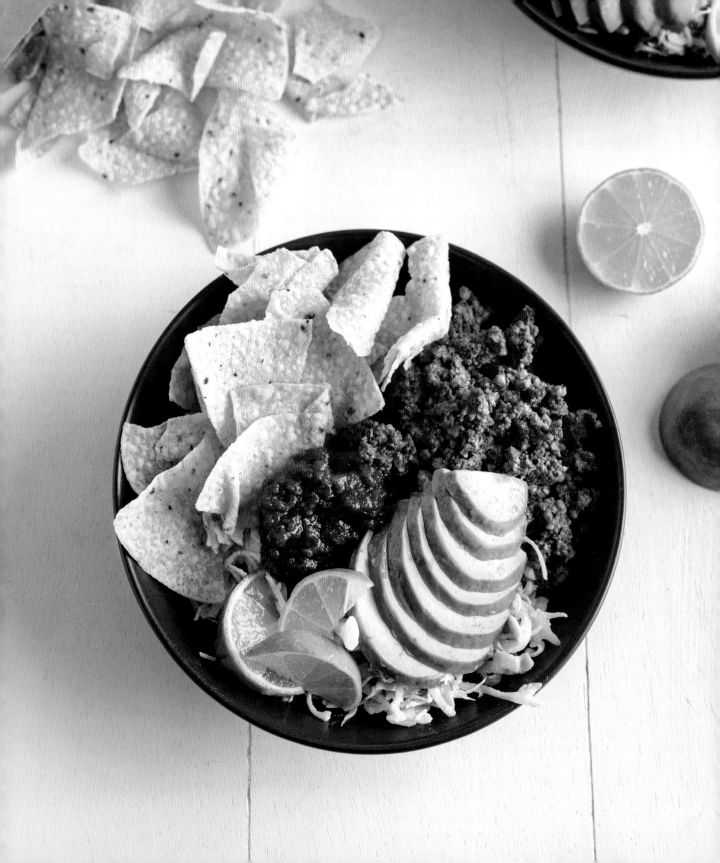

The Best Damn Taco Salad

While growing up, I lived for the taco salad from Taco Bell. And while that will always be tasty and have a place in my heart, I am all about making elevated versions at home. The jalapeño-sunflower crema might be one of the most delicious things I have ever tasted. (It also makes an amazing mayo substitution on pretty much any kind of sandwich, grilled cheese included . . . just saying.) Mix that all together with the perfectly spiced walnut meat and fresh crunchy vegetables, and you have a filling and satisfying salad. It's anything but bland or boring!

SERVES 4

JALAPEÑO-SUNFLOWER CREMA

1 cup (145 g) raw sunflower seeds, soaked in very hot water for 15 minutes (see Note)

½ cup plus 1 tbsp (135 ml) water, plus more if needed

¼ cup (60 ml) fresh lime juice

1 tsp garlic powder

½ jalapeño pepper

Salt

SALAD

1 large cabbage, shredded on a mandoline (preferred) or thinly sliced

1 cup (100 g) sliced green onion

1 cup (40 g) loosely packed fresh cilantro leaves

½ cup (80 g) sliced red onion

1 cup (260 g) salsa

1 ripe avocado, sliced

1 prepared recipe Walnut Taco Meat (page 42)

GARNISHES

Vegan tortilla chips

Lime wedges

Make the crema: Rinse and drain the soaked sunflower seeds. In a blender, combine the sunflower seeds, fresh water, lime juice, garlic powder, jalapeño and salt to taste. Blend on high speed until smooth. Taste and adjust, adding more salt to bring out the flavors and more water if you prefer a thinner dressing.

Make the salad: In a large bowl, combine the shredded cabbage, green onion, cilantro and red onion and toss well. Add the jalapeño crema and toss well to evenly coat the mixture. Divide equally among 4 serving bowls. Top each bowl with the salsa, avocado slices and walnut taco meat. Garnish with tortilla chips and lime wedges and serve immediately.

If making ahead, mix everything as written, except the avocado, which should be added just before serving. Store the dressing and walnut taco meat separately, until ready to eat. Everything will keep well in airtight containers in the fridge for up to a week.

Note: *If you do not have a high-speed blender, soak your sunflower seeds for up to an hour, to protect your blender.*

Spring Vegetable Panzanella

Being predominately of Italian descent, I am no stranger to panzanella, a traditional salad that contains soaked stale bread and tomatoes. It's a great way to use up day-old loaves. Inspired by the classic but adding my own spin, I combined fresh springtime vegetables, including asparagus, green peas and sugar snaps with a bright, lovely pesto that will leave you wanting more. The sweetness is balanced out by the peppery arugula and tied together with the avocado and bread. This is amazing for a beautiful spring afternoon in the park and makes a great picnic or potluck dish as well!

SERVES 4

MIXED HERB PESTO

½ cup (67 g) raw pine nuts

3 cloves garlic

1¼ cups (52 g) tightly packed fresh basil leaves

½ cup (21 g) tightly packed fresh mint leaves

½ cup (31 g) tightly packed fresh parsley or (21 g) cilantro leaves

3 tbsp (45 ml) fresh lemon juice

½ cup (120 ml) avocado oil

Salt and freshly ground black pepper

SALAD

12 oz (340 g) asparagus spears, preferably thick stalks

20 oz (567 g) sugar snap peas

3 cups (150 g) cubed vegan bread

¾ cup (113 g) sweet peas

½ cup (58 g) chopped watermelon radish (preferred) or purple or red radish

3 cups (65 g) tightly packed arugula

2 cups (63 g) tightly packed spinach

1 ripe avocado, diced

Preheat the oven to 450°F (230°C).

Make the pesto: In a food processor fitted with an S blade, combine the pine nuts and garlic. Pulse in 10-second bursts, 3 times, or until a crumble is formed. Add the fresh herbs and lemon juice and pulse again in 10-second bursts, 3 times, stopping to scrape down the sides, if needed. With the processor on low speed, slowly drizzle in the avocado oil through the center of the lid. Add salt and pepper to taste; I use about 1 teaspoon of each. Set aside.

Make the salad: Bring a medium-sized pot of water to a boil. Meanwhile, create an ice bath by putting ice cubes in a large bowl of water; set the ice bath aside. Blanch the asparagus by adding the spears to the boiling water and cooking for 2 to 3 minutes (if your spears are on the thinner side, blanch for only 1 to 2 minutes). Transfer the asparagus to the ice bath to stop the cooking process.

Repeat this process for the sugar snap peas, blanching for 1 to 2 minutes. Let both the asparagus and sugar snap peas sit in the ice bath for at least 5 minutes each. Then, drain the water and pat dry both veggies with a paper towel or clean dish towel. Cut the asparagus into 1-inch (2.5-cm) lengths and the sugar snap peas in half horizontally.

Meanwhile, lay the cubed bread in a single layer on a baking sheet and heat in the oven for 5 to 8 minutes, or until lightly toasted. Set aside.

In a large bowl, combine the asparagus, sugar snap peas, sweet peas, radish, arugula, spinach, avocado, bread and pesto. Mix well to evenly coat everything with the pesto. Let the salad rest for 10 minutes so the bread has some time to soak up some of the pesto. Then, divide equally among 4 serving bowls and serve.

If making ahead, prepare everything as directed, except the avocado, which should be added just before serving, and store in an airtight container in the fridge for up to 5 days.

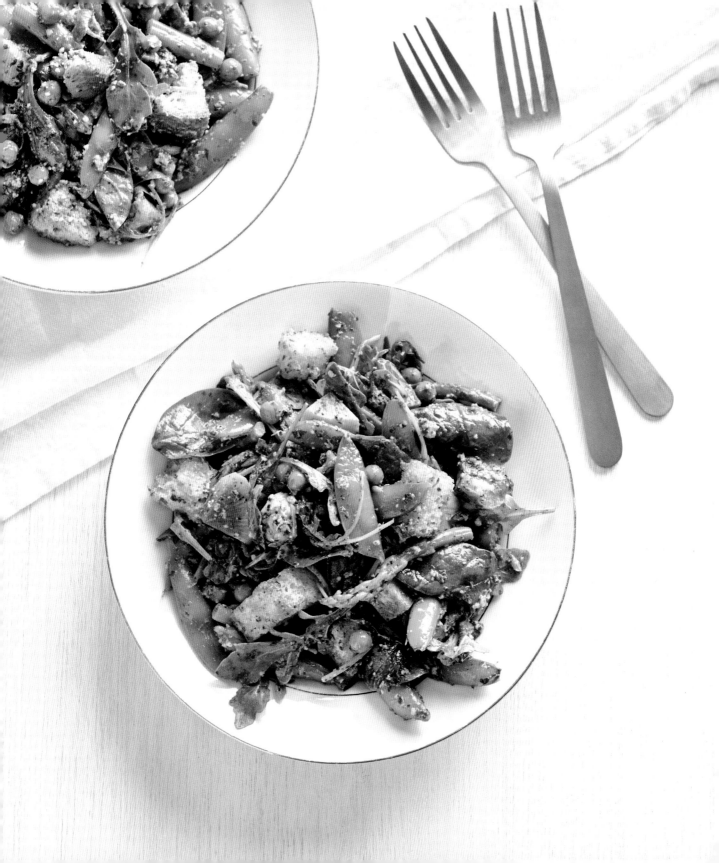

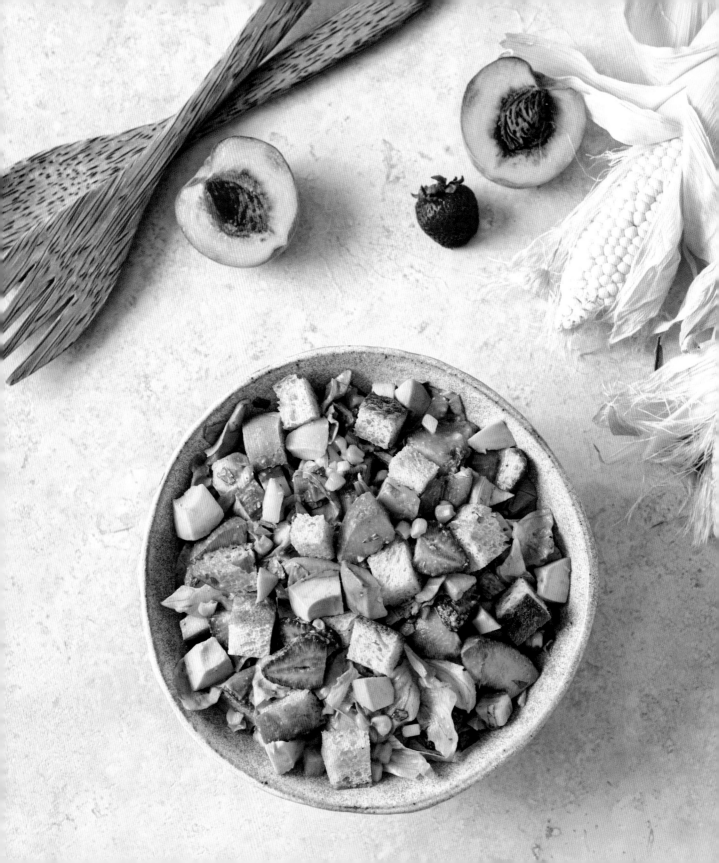

Summer Vegetable Panzanella

There are several reasons why I love living in Southern California. The abundance of produce is at the top of the list right behind the gorgeous weather. This beautiful panzanella really shines with the juicy, sweet peaches and strawberries, balanced out with perfectly spiced corn and creamy avocados. Bonus points if you can get your hands on California avocados—their flavor is unmatched. The mint really pops against the savory dressing and the cucumber adds a lovely crunchy element. This is perfect for a backyard barbecue or Sunday brunch with mimosas!

SERVES 4 AS MAIN

ZIPPY TAHINI DRESSING

½ cup (120 ml) olive oil

⅓ cup (80 ml) apple cider vinegar

¼ cup (60 g) tahini

¼ cup (60 ml) coconut aminos (preferred), tamari or soy sauce

1 tsp garlic powder

½ tsp crushed red pepper flakes

Salt and freshly ground black pepper

3 cups (150 g) cubed vegan bread

CORN

2 ears corn, shucked (see Note)

2 tbsp (30 ml) melted vegan butter

1 tsp garlic powder

½ tsp ground cumin

⅛ tsp cayenne pepper

Salt and freshly ground black pepper

SALAD

2 heads butter lettuce, roughly chopped

3 cups (510 g) hulled and sliced strawberries

2 medium-sized ripe peaches, pitted and chopped into bite-sized pieces

1 English cucumber, diced

1 cup (42 g) tightly packed, roughly chopped fresh mint

2 ripe avocados, peeled, pitted and cubed

Preheat the oven to 450°F (230°C).

Make the dressing: In a blender, add the olive oil, vinegar, tahini, coconut aminos, garlic powder and red pepper flakes and blend on high to combine. Add salt and black pepper to taste. Set aside.

Make the corn: Bring a medium-sized pot of water to a boil, then add the corn and cook for 10 minutes.

Lay the cubed bread in a single layer on a baking sheet and heat in the oven for 5 to 8 minutes until lightly toasted. When done, set aside.

When the corn is ready, transfer the ears to a bowl to keep the kernels from flying everywhere, then use a sharp knife to carefully slice off the kernels. Discard the cobs. Add the melted butter, garlic powder, cumin, cayenne, salt and black pepper to taste and toss the kernels to evenly coat. Set aside.

Make the salad: In a large bowl, combine the lettuce, strawberries, peaches, cucumber, mint, corn kernels, bread and half of the avocado cubes. Add the dressing and toss to evenly coat. Let the salad rest for 10 minutes, giving the bread some time to soak up the dressing. Then, divide equally among 4 serving bowls and top each with the remaining avocado.

If making this ahead of time, mix everything as directed, except the avocado, which should be added just before serving. Store the dressing separately until ready to serve and keep everything else in an airtight container in the fridge for up to 5 days.

Note: I also enjoy cooking corn in a skillet! If you'd like to try it that way, in a medium-sized lidded skillet, melt the butter over medium heat. Add the husked ears of corn. Cover and cook, turning the corn every 5 or so minutes, for 20 to 25 minutes, or until all sides of the ears are cooked. Remove from the heat and proceed with the recipe.

Autumn Vegetable Panzanella

Keeping on with the panzanella vibes, this one incorporates beautiful fall flavors and ingredients. The sweet yet savory creamy tahini pairs perfectly with the broccoli and Brussels sprouts. It is made a complete and filling meal with the spinach, bread and pistachios. This easy and delicious dish will likely be on repeat all autumn long!

SERVES 2

MAPLE TAHINI DRESSING

⅓ cup (80 g) tahini

¼ cup (60 ml) water

1 tbsp (15 ml) pure maple syrup

¼ tsp garlic powder

Salt and freshly ground black pepper

SALAD

1½ cups (75 g) cubed vegan bread

2 cups (142 g) broccoli florets

3 cups (264 g) Brussels sprouts, cut in half

¼ cup (60 ml) melted coconut oil

Salt and freshly ground black pepper

2 cups (65 g) tightly packed baby spinach

⅓ cup (41 g) pistachios

Preheat the oven to 450°F (230°C).

Make the dressing: In a small bowl, vigorously whisk together the tahini, water, maple syrup and garlic powder to combine, then add salt and pepper to taste. Set aside.

Make the salad: Lay out the cubed bread in a single layer on a baking sheet and heat in the oven for 5 to 8 minutes, or until lightly toasted. Remove from the oven and set aside, transferring to a bowl if necessary to free up the baking sheet for the next step.

Lay out the broccoli florets and Brussels sprouts in a single layer on 1 or 2 baking sheets. Cover evenly with the melted coconut oil, sprinkle with salt and pepper to taste, toss to coat and then roast in the oven for 12 to 14 minutes, or until tender and turning brown. Remove from the oven and set aside.

In a large bowl, combine the spinach, bread, roasted veggies and dressing. Toss to coat and mix well, then divide among 4 serving bowls and top evenly with the pistachios.

If making this ahead of time, mix everything as described. Store the dressing separately until ready to serve and keep everything else in an airtight container in the fridge for up to 5 days.

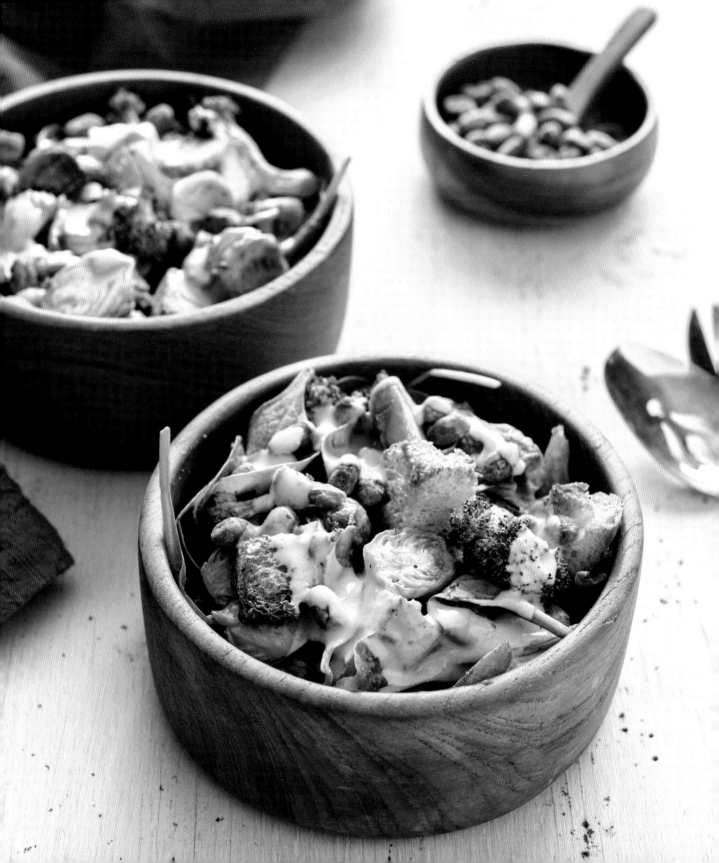

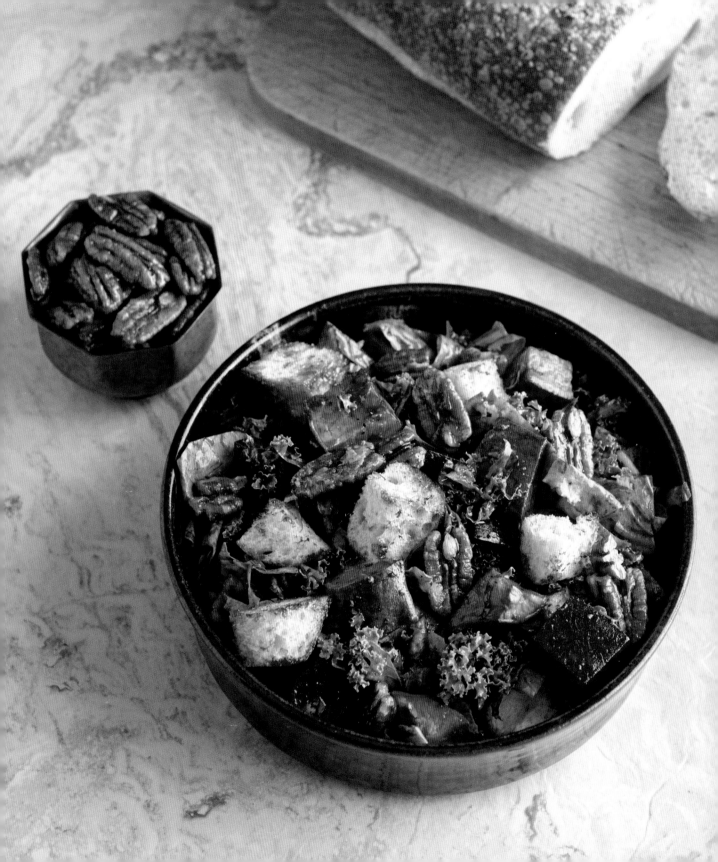

Winter Vegetable Panzanella

To finish out this panzanella trend, I brought together some of my favorite seasonal ingredients for this winter version. I love the nuttiness that the walnut oil adds to this salad; it is subtly sweet, which pairs well with the balsamic vinegar. The grounding root vegetables and toasted bread make this salad incredibly satisfying, while the kale and romaine up the nutritional value. For some extra fun, it's topped off with some candied pecans—which make any salad more delicious!

SERVES 2

WALNUT VINAIGRETTE DRESSING

¾ cup (175 ml) toasted or roasted walnut oil

⅓ cup (80 ml) balsamic vinegar

2 tsp (10 ml) pure maple syrup

2 tsp (10 ml) Dijon mustard

1 tsp garlic powder

Salt and freshly ground black pepper

SALAD

1½ cups (75 g) cubed vegan bread

3 cups (400 g) cubed sweet potato (1" [2.5-cm] cubes)

2 tbsp (30 ml) melted coconut oil

Salt and freshly ground pepper

3 cups (208 g) tightly packed chopped kale leaves

2 cups (32 g) tightly packed chopped romaine

2 cups (450 g) cubed roasted beets (1" [2.5-cm] cubes) (see Note)

½ cup (56 g) candied pecans

Preheat the oven to 450°F (230°C).

Make the dressing: In a blender, combine the walnut oil, balsamic vinegar, tahini, maple syrup, Dijon and garlic powder. Starting on low speed, slowly increase the speed to high and blend for 30 seconds, or until emulsified. Then, add salt and pepper to taste. Set aside.

Make the salad: Lay out the cubed bread in a single layer on a baking sheet and heat in the oven for 5 to 8 minutes, or until lightly toasted. Remove from the oven and set aside, transferring to a bowl if necessary to free up the baking sheet for the next step.

Lay out the sweet potato cubes in a single layer on a baking sheet. Add the coconut oil and season with salt and pepper. Toss well to evenly coat and then roast in the oven for 12 to 15 minutes, or until fork-tender and turning brown. Remove from the oven and set aside.

In a large bowl, combine the kale leaves and half of the dressing. Using tongs, massage the kale with the dressing to soften the leaves for about 1 minute. Add the romaine, roasted beets, sweet potato, bread and desired amount of dressing. Toss well and let rest for 10 minutes. Then, divide equally among 2 serving bowls and top with the candied pecans. Enjoy!

If making ahead of time, mix everything as written, except the dressing which should be reserved until ready to serve. Store everything in airtight containers in the fridge for up to a week.

Note: To save time when making this recipe, use prepared store-bought roasted beets. If you want to make them from scratch, see the directions on page 70.

Cauli-Ranch Salad

There is so much to love about this salad! The ranch dressing is herbaceous and flavorful while adding additional creaminess alongside the avocado. The barbecued cauliflower pretty much speaks for itself here, with its tangy sweetness that goes so well with the spiced corn, tomatoes and black beans. This salad will surely have you coming back for more!

SERVES 4

SUNFLOWER RANCH DRESSING

1 cup (145 g) raw sunflower seeds, soaked with very hot water for 15 minutes (see Note)

1 cup (240 ml) unsweetened almond milk

3 tbsp (45 ml) fresh lemon juice

2 cloves garlic

1 tsp onion powder

2 tsp (10 ml) apple cider vinegar

¼ cup (60 ml) avocado or grapeseed oil

2 tbsp (6 g) tightly packed minced fresh dill

Salt and freshly ground black pepper

BBQ CAULI

2 tsp (10 ml) avocado oil

6 heaping cups (600 g) bite-sized cauliflower florets

¾ cup (188 g) barbecue sauce, divided

SALAD

1 cup (180 g) diced tomato

1 cup (150 g) corn kernels

1 (15-oz [425-g]) can black beans, drained and rinsed

1 tsp ground cumin

2 tsp (5 g) chili powder

2 tsp (6 g) garlic powder

8 to 10 cups (440 to 550 g) chopped romaine lettuce

1 to 2 ripe avocados, diced

½ cup (80 g) thinly sliced red onion

½ cup (21 g) tightly packed chopped fresh cilantro

Make the dressing: Rinse and drain the sunflower seeds and place them in a high-speed blender along with the almond milk, lemon juice, garlic, onion powder and vinegar. Blend on high speed for 1 to 2 minutes, or until smooth and creamy, stopping to scrape down the sides or use the tamper to help, if needed. While the motor is running, slowly add the avocado oil through the center of the lid until emulsified. Transfer to a bowl, add the dill and mix well. Add salt and pepper to taste. Set aside.

Make the cauliflower: Preheat the oven to 450°F (230°C). Coat a baking sheet with the avocado oil. Add the cauliflower and ½ cup (125 g) of the barbecue sauce to the prepared pan. Using your hands or a spatula, mix well to evenly coat the florets with the sauce. Roast in the oven for 15 to 20 minutes, stopping to toss halfway through. Remove from the oven and let cool for 5 minutes, then add the remaining ¼ cup (63 g) of barbecue sauce, toss to coat and set aside.

Make the salad: In a small bowl, combine the tomato, corn, black beans, cumin, chili powder and garlic powder and mix well. Set aside.

In a large bowl, combine the chopped romaine and ½ to ¾ cup (120 to 175 ml) of the dressing. Mix well to evenly coat and then add more dressing, if desired. You will likely have some dressing left over. Divide up the salad greens equally among 4 serving bowls and top each bowl equally with the tomato mixture. Top each bowl with avocado, cauliflower, red onion and fresh cilantro. Serve immediately.

If making ahead, mix everything together as directed, except the dressing and avocado, which should be added just before serving. Store the salad in individual servings or 1 large airtight container in the fridge for up to a week.

Note: *If you do not have a high-speed blender, soak your sunflower seeds for up to an hour or overnight, to protect your blender.*

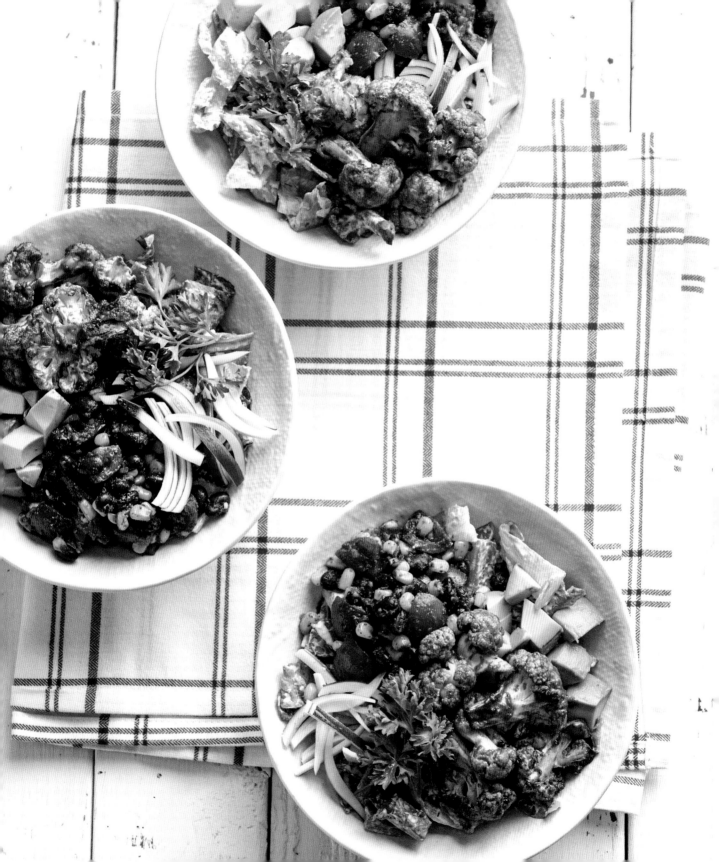

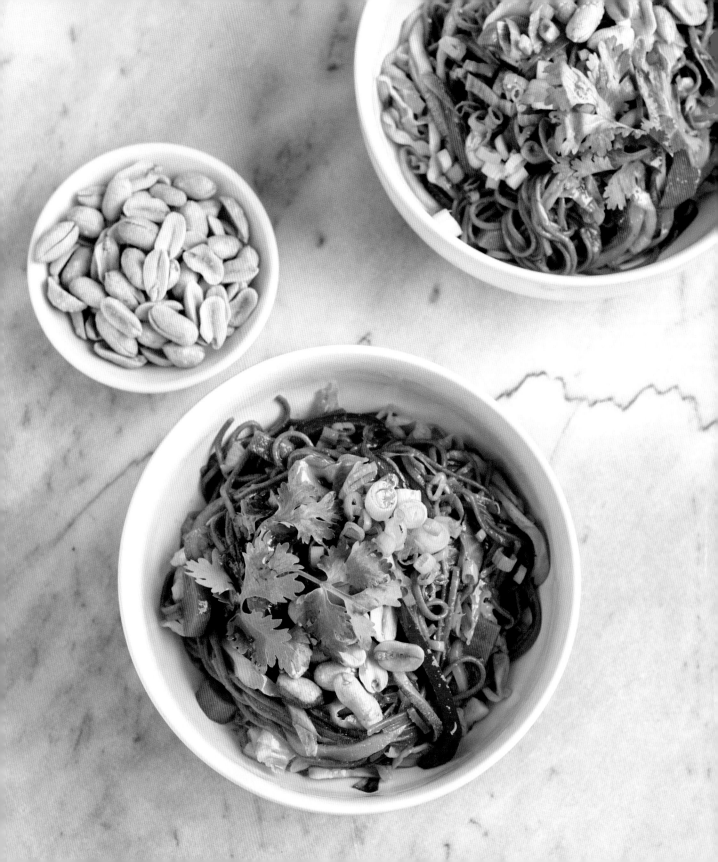

Thai-a-Knot Salad

Is it still a salad if it's warm? I think that's possible, and if someone somewhere has a rule that all salads must be cold, well, please pass along that I broke the rule and I'm feeling good about being a rebel! And if you make this dish you might feel pretty good about it, too. The sesame sauce is delicious. It's sweet, nutty, spicy, savory . . . what's not to like? The vegetables are crunchy, while the noodles are extra comforting. Everything is brought together with toppings like cilantro, peanuts and green onion!

SERVES 4

SESAME SAUCE

¾ cup (175 ml) toasted sesame oil

¼ cup (60 ml) soy sauce or tamari

2 tbsp (30 ml) coconut aminos

3 tbsp (45 ml) pure maple syrup

2 tbsp (30 ml) sriracha

2 tsp (6 g) garlic powder

NOODLES

9 oz (255 g) dried soba noodles

SALAD

2 tbsp (28 g) coconut oil

1 red bell pepper, seeded and thinly sliced

2 medium-sized carrots, peeled and chopped

Salt and freshly ground black pepper

1 small green cabbage, thinly sliced

3 medium-sized zucchini, spiralized into noodles

½ cup (20 g) loosely packed chopped fresh basil (optional)

GARNISHES

Fresh cilantro

Peanuts

Green onion

Make the sauce: In a small bowl, whisk together the toasted sesame oil, soy sauce, coconut aminos, maple syrup, sriracha and garlic powder until well combined. Taste and see whether you want to adjust any of the seasonings.

Make the noodles: Bring a medium-sized pot of water to a boil, then cook the noodles according to the package instructions. Drain and rinse in cold water, then transfer to a large bowl and mix in one-quarter of the sauce to prevent the noodles from sticking. Set aside.

Make the salad: In a large skillet or wok, melt the coconut oil over medium heat. Once hot, add the bell pepper and carrots. Cook for 5 to 6 minutes and season with salt and pepper to taste. Add the sliced cabbage and cook for another 2 to 3 minutes, stirring occasionally. Add the zucchini noodles and cook, stirring occasionally, for 5 to 6 minutes or until softened.

Remove from the heat and, using tongs or a slotted spoon—leaving as much cooking liquid as possible in the skillet so it doesn't water down the salad—transfer the veggie mixture to the bowl of noodles. Add the basil (if using) and remaining sauce and mix well. Divide equally among 4 serving bowls and garnish with cilantro, peanuts and green onion. Serve immediately.

If making ahead of time, mix everything as written, except reserve the sauce until ready to serve. It should be stored separately. Keep everything in airtight containers in the fridge for 4 to 5 days.

Farmers' Market Chopped Salad

Something that I pride myself on a little bit is being able to make a delicious salad that is filling and flavorful. This one certainly fits the bill. The roasted root vegetables are so grounding paired with the fresh mixed greens and refreshing cucumber, while the avocado and quinoa make it a substantial salad. Topped off with microgreens, hemp seeds and almonds, it's a nutritional powerhouse!

SERVES 4

ROASTED VEGGIES

4 medium-sized beets

¼ cup (60 ml) balsamic vinegar

2 cups (266 g) cubed sweet potato (1" [2.5-cm] cubes)

2 tbsp (30 ml) melted coconut oil

½ tsp garlic powder

½ tsp dried rosemary

½ tsp smoked paprika

Salt and freshly ground black pepper

BALSAMIC VINAIGRETTE

⅓ cup (80 ml) balsamic vinegar

1 tbsp (15 ml) Dijon mustard

1 tbsp (15 ml) pure maple syrup

1 cup (240 ml) olive oil

2 tsp (6 g) garlic powder

2 tsp (2 g) dried oregano

Pink salt and black pepper to taste

SALAD

4 cups (220 g) chopped romaine lettuce

4 cups (120 g) loosely packed baby spinach

2 cups (370 g) cooked white quinoa

2 cups (270 g) diced cucumber

2 ripe avocados, diced

GARNISHES

Microgreens

Hemp seeds

Chopped roasted and salted almonds

Roast the veggies: Preheat the oven to 450°F (230°C).

Wash the beets, then pat dry and wrap them up in foil to form a pouch. Roast in the oven for 45 minutes to 1 hour, or until soft and easily pierced with a fork. Remove from the oven and let cool for 5 minutes, then peel and cut into 1-inch (2.5-cm) cubes. Transfer to a small bowl, add the vinegar, mix well and then set aside to marinate.

Place the sweet potato on a baking sheet, top with the melted coconut oil, then add the garlic powder, rosemary, smoked paprika and a generous pinch of salt and pepper. Mix well to evenly coat. Then, spread out in a single layer and roast for 12 to 15 minutes, or until fork-tender. Remove from the oven and set aside.

Make the vinaigrette: In a small bowl, combine the vinegar, Dijon and maple syrup, then slowly whisk in the olive oil to emulsify. Add the garlic powder, oregano, pink salt and pepper to taste and mix well again. Set aside.

Make the salad: In a large bowl, toss together the romaine and spinach. Add the quinoa, cucumber, avocados, sweet potato and beets and toss again. Add the dressing and mix well. Divide equally among 4 serving plates, then garnish with microgreens, hemp seeds and almonds. Serve immediately.

If making ahead, mix everything as directed except the dressing, which should be added just before serving. Store the salad in individual servings or 1 large airtight container in the fridge for up to a week.

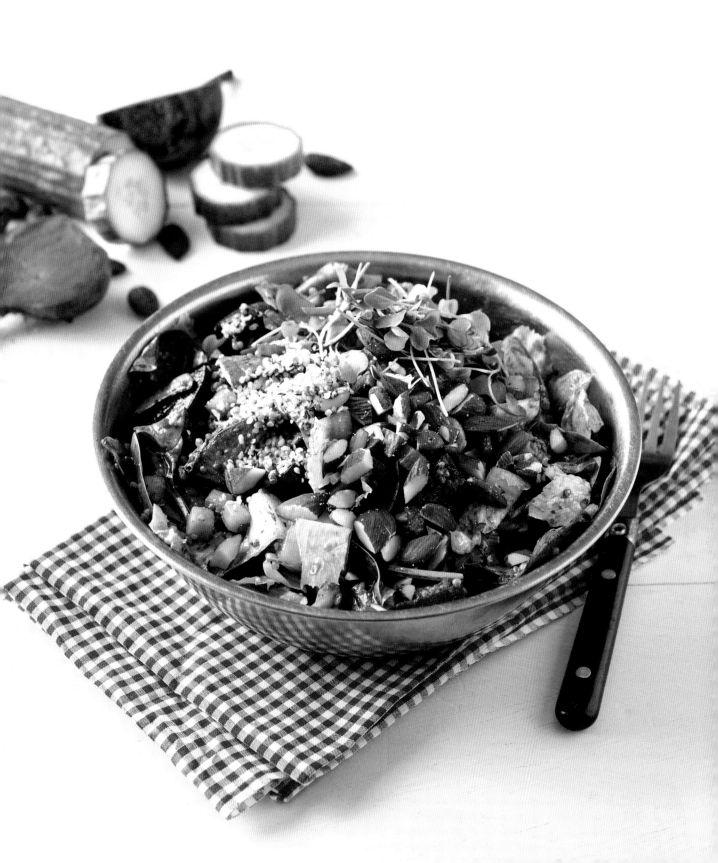

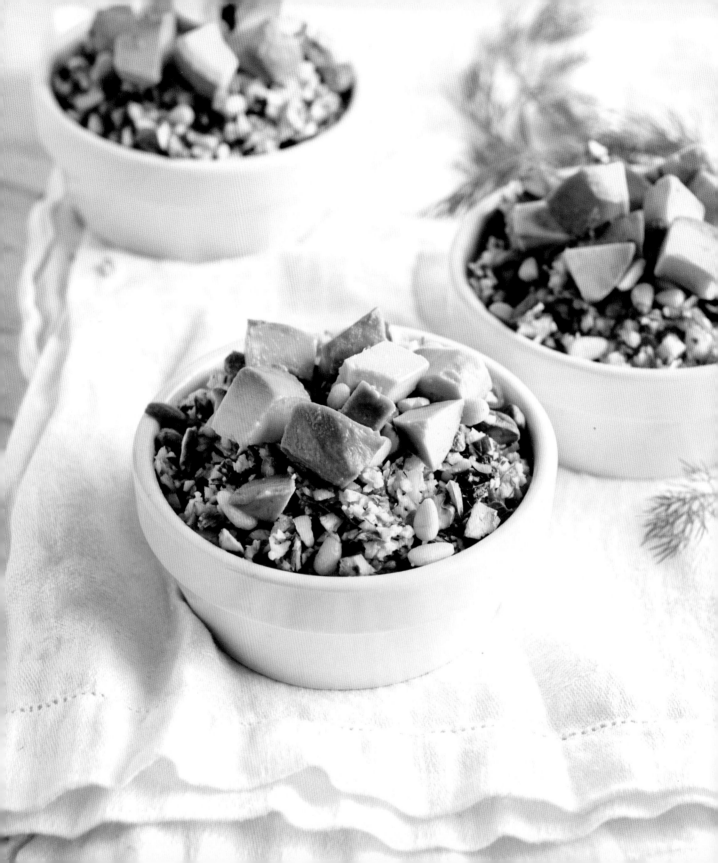

Mixed Herb Tabbouleh

This is a ridiculously fun and fresh take on traditional tabbouleh salad inspired by a talented chef named Nicole Dayani in Los Angeles. If you're ever in Beverly Hills, I highly recommend taking a cooking class of hers. It will be a night you will never forget. What I love is how she is always taking classic recipes and updating them with a modern twist. Since cauliflower rice has been a recent phenomenon in the health and wellness world, it made sense to use it here and to bring in an extra sweet element, so I added parsnip rice, too. Paired with the variety of fresh herbs, umami-rich sun-dried tomatoes and crispy, crunchy radish and nuts, each bite is a serious VIP mouth party. Obviously, I added avocado, and this is officially an over-the-top delicious salad.

----------------- SERVES 6 AS A SIDE -----------------

VIBRANT VINAIGRETTE

¼ cup (60 ml) fresh lemon juice

¼ cup (60 ml) red wine vinegar

1 tsp garlic powder

¾ cup (175 ml) olive oil

SALAD

6 cups (600 g) riced cauliflower

2 cups (200 g) riced parsnip (see Note)

3 cups (180 g) loosely packed finely chopped fresh parsley leaves

3 cups (120 g) loosely packed finely chopped fresh cilantro leaves

1 cup (60 g) loosely packed fresh dill leaves

1 cup (100 g) loosely packed finely chopped green onion

1 cup (40 g) loosely packed finely chopped fresh basil leaves

1 cup (110 g) chopped oil-packed sun-dried tomatoes

½ cup (58 g) finely chopped radish

GARNISHES

½ cup (62 g) chopped pistachios

½ cup (67 g) pine nuts

2 avocados, diced

Pink salt

Make the vinaigrette: In a small bowl, combine the lemon juice, vinegar and garlic powder. Mix well, then whisk in the olive oil until emulsified. Set aside.

Make the salad: In a large bowl, combine the cauliflower rice, parsnip rice, parsley, cilantro, dill, green onion, basil, sun-dried tomatoes and radish. Mix well, then add the dressing and toss to coat.

Divide equally among 6 serving bowls and top each bowl with the pistachios, pine nuts and avocado. Add pink salt to taste. Serve immediately.

If making ahead, mix everything as directed except the dressing and avocado, which should be added just before serving. Store in individual servings or 1 large airtight container in the fridge for up to a week.

Note: *To make the parsnip rice, peel off the skin with a vegetable peeler. Then, using a knife, finely dice until the result resembles cauliflower rice. Alternatively, you could use a food processor, fitted with the cheese grater attachment, to chop into ricelike pieces.*

Ginger Soba Noodle Salad

I'll admit that I have always found it a little funny to call a cold bowl of noodles a salad simply because it's cold, but here I am . . . calling a cold bowl of noodles a salad! Oh well! The ginger vinaigrette will make your taste buds do a little dance, and it totally brings out the deliciousness of the sugar snap peas, noodles and radish. The spinach, mint and cilantro add an additional layer of flavor that sends it over the top.

SERVES 4

GINGER VINAIGRETTE

¼ cup (60 ml) rice vinegar

3 tbsp (45 ml) fresh lime juice

1 (1" [2.5-cm]) knob fresh ginger, grated (preferred) or minced

1 jalapeño pepper, stemmed, halved lengthwise, seeded if desired and finely chopped

1 tbsp (15 ml) pure maple syrup or agave nectar

1 tsp Dijon mustard

¾ cup (175 ml) avocado or grapeseed oil (olive oil not recommended)

Salt and freshly ground black pepper

VEGGIES & NOODLES

10 oz (280 g) sugar snap peas

9 oz (255 g) soba noodles

1 tsp sesame oil

½ cup (58 g) thinly sliced and chopped watermelon radish or red or purple radish

⅓ cup (14 g) tightly packed chopped fresh mint

⅓ cup (14 g) tightly packed chopped fresh cilantro

2 green onions, sliced

4 cups (130 g) tightly packed baby spinach or watercress

GARNISHES

Sesame seeds

Green onion

Make the vinaigrette: In a small bowl, whisk together the vinegar, lime juice, ginger, jalapeño, maple syrup and Dijon. Then, slowly whisk in the avocado oil. Season with salt and pepper to taste, then set aside.

Make the vegetables and noodles: In a medium-sized bowl, combine ice cubes and cold water to make an ice bath and set aside. Bring a medium-sized pot of salted water to a boil. Add the snap peas to the boiling water and boil for 1 to 2 minutes, then transfer to the ice bath to stop the cooking.

Keep the pot of water on the stove to reuse for the noodles. Bring the water back to a boil and cook the noodles according to the package instructions. Drain and rinse with cold water, then transfer to a bowl and add the sesame oil, mixing well to keep the noodles from sticking.

Drain the ice water from the sugar snap peas, pat them dry with a towel and add them to the bowl of noodles, then add the watermelon radish, mint, cilantro and green onions. Add two-thirds of the dressing and mix well.

Divide the spinach equally among 4 bowls, drizzle with the rest of the dressing, then divide the noodle mixture and place on top. Garnish with sesame seeds and green onion, then serve.

If making ahead of time, mix everything as directed except the dressing, which should be added just before serving. Store the salad in individual servings or 1 large airtight container in the fridge for up to a week.

Note: For extra crunch, add some chopped peanuts.

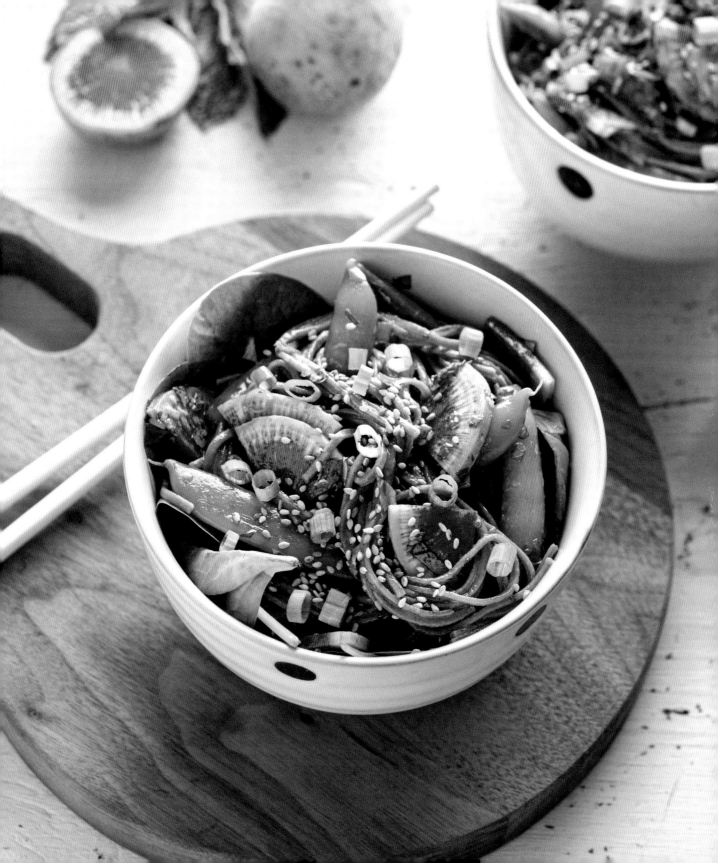

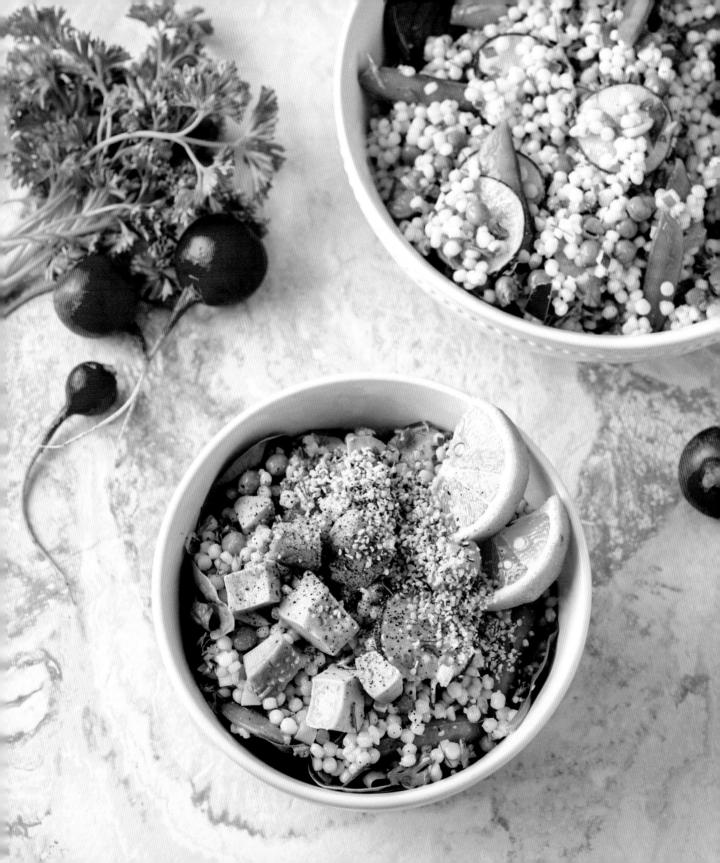

Kiss Kiss Couscous

If the classic macaroni salad had a bougie relative, it would be this salad. Israeli couscous is pretty much the same thing as a macaroni noodle but shaped like a teeny tiny ball. When paired with sweet and crunchy sugar snap peas, green peas and radish, then mixed with an assortment of fresh herbs, then coated with a simple yet vibrant vinaigrette and finished with avocado, hemp seeds and lemon wedges, it's an elevated and fancy-ass version. You can't help but raise a pinkie when eating.

SERVES 4

COUSCOUS
2 tbsp (30 ml) avocado oil

3 cups (525 g) dried Israeli couscous

4½ cups (1.1 L) warm water (about 110°F [43°C])

Salt

SIMPLE VINAIGRETTE
⅓ cup (80 ml) red wine vinegar

3 cloves garlic, minced

2 tbsp (30 ml) pure maple syrup

1 cup (240 ml) olive oil

Salt and freshly ground black pepper

SALAD
10 oz (280 g) sugar snap peas

2 cups (260 g) frozen sweet peas

1 cup (116 g) thinly sliced radish

1½ cups (75 g) finely chopped, tightly packed fresh herbs (see Notes)

½ cup (80 g) finely diced red onion

2 green onions, chopped

1 tbsp (9 g) garlic powder

8 cups (240 g) baby spinach leaves

2 avocados, cubed

Salt and freshly ground black pepper

GARNISHES
Lemon wedges

Hemp seeds

Make the couscous: In a medium-sized saucepan, heat the avocado oil over medium heat. Once hot, add the couscous and stir for 30 seconds. Then, add the warm water and salt and bring to a boil. Cover, lower the heat to medium and cook until all the water is absorbed, about 12 minutes. Drain and rinse with cool water, then set aside.

Meanwhile, make the vinaigrette: In a small bowl, combine the vinegar, garlic and maple syrup, then slowly whisk in the olive oil until emulsified. Season with salt and pepper to taste. Set aside.

In a medium-sized bowl, create an ice bath with ice cubes and cold water and set aside. Bring a medium-sized pot of water to a boil. Add the snap peas to the boiling water and boil for 3 minutes, then transfer to the ice bath to stop the cooking.

Defrost the sweet peas according to their package directions.

In a large bowl, combine the radish, fresh herbs, red onion, green onions, garlic powder, sweet peas, sugar snap peas and cooked couscous. Add three-quarters of the dressing and mix well.

To serve, divide the spinach equally among 4 serving bowls and drizzle each with some of the remaining dressing. Add a layer of the couscous mixture. Divide the avocado among the bowls, season with salt and pepper to taste, garnish with lemon wedges and hemp seeds and serve.

If making ahead of time, mix everything together as directed, except the avocado, which should be added just before serving, and store in an airtight container in the fridge for up to a week.

Notes: *For the fresh herbs, I recommend a mix of at least two of the following, but up to all four: cilantro, mint, dill or parsley.*

For additional crunch, add some dry toasted slivered almonds.

Topanga Chopped Salad

This salad is just so good and so simple. It got its unique name because I made it for a retreat that took place in Topanga Canyon, California, which, if you don't know, is an absolutely beautiful place worthy of absolutely delicious salads! At first glance, this is a classic chopped salad, nothing too fancy. It has a great combination of cucumber, tomatoes, garbanzo beans and olives, but what makes it extra special are the fresh herbs and za'atar. They add so much flavor and complexity to each bite and the simple za'atar vinaigrette really makes it all shine.

--- SERVES 4 ---

ZA'ATAR VINAIGRETTE

¼ cup (60 ml) fresh lemon juice

¾ cup (175 ml) olive or avocado oil

1 tsp za'atar, plus more to taste

1 tsp garlic powder

Salt and freshly ground black pepper

SALAD

10 cups (550 g) chopped romaine lettuce

1 English cucumber, cut into thin half-moons

3 Roma tomatoes, cut into bite-size pieces

1 (15-oz [425-g]) can garbanzo beans (chickpeas), drained and rinsed

1 cup (100 g) pitted and halved Kalamata olives

½ cup (80 g) thinly sliced red onion

½ cup (20 g) chopped fresh mint

½ cup (30 g) chopped fresh parsley

½ cup (20 g) chopped fresh cilantro

3 green onions, sliced

1 to 2 avocados, diced

2 tsp (5 g) za'atar, plus more for topping (optional)

GARNISHES

Microgreens

Chopped cashews

Make the vinaigrette: Pour the lemon juice into a medium-sized bowl, slowly whisk in the oil, then whisk vigorously until combined. Add the za'atar, garlic powder and salt and pepper to taste, whisk again and set aside.

Make the salad: In a large salad bowl, combine the chopped romaine and three-quarters each of the cucumber, tomatoes, garbanzo beans, olives, red onion, mint, parsley, cilantro, green onions and avocado. Add three-quarters of the dressing as well as the za'atar. Toss everything to mix and evenly coat. Then, add the remaining salad ingredients on top and pour the remaining dressing. Garnish with microgreens, chopped cashews and additional za'atar, if desired. Serve immediately.

If making ahead of time, mix everything as directed, except the avocado, which should be added just before serving, and store the dressing separately from everything else until ready to serve.

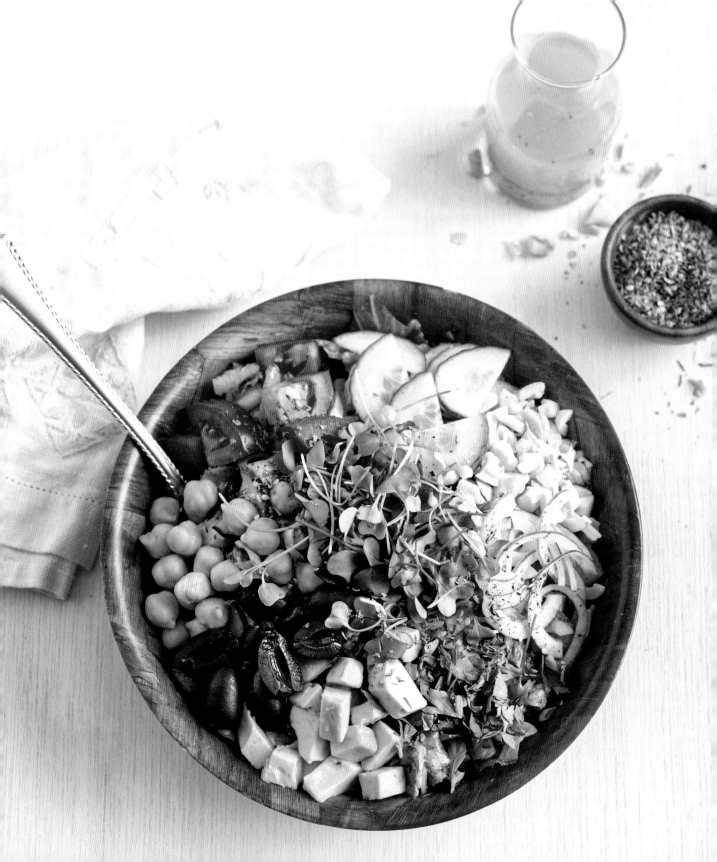

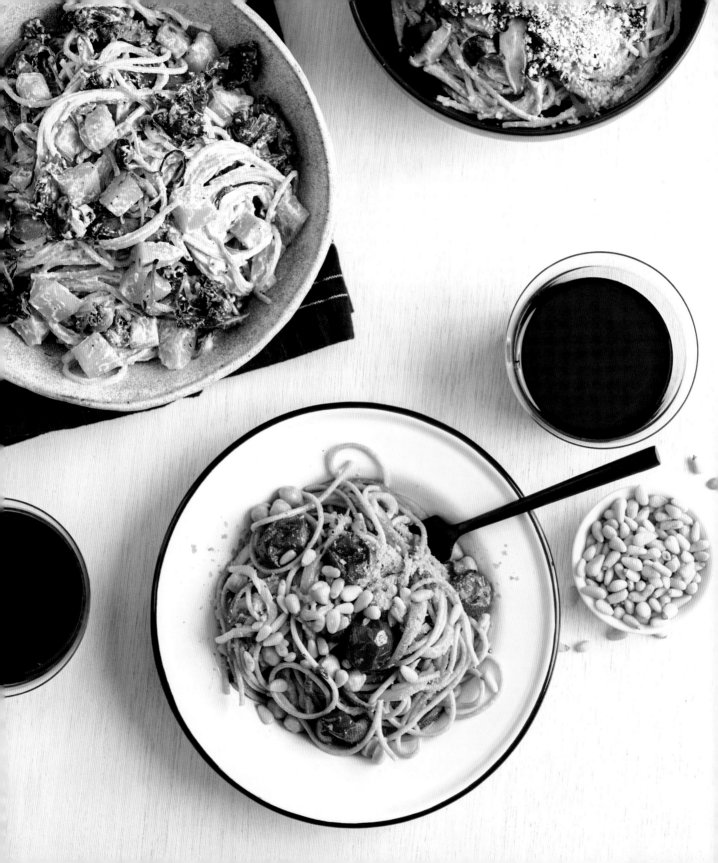

Comforting, Veggie-Rich Pasta Bowls

Years ago, when I was just entering recovery from my eating disorder and discovering plant-based diets, I read several books, including *The China Study*, by T. Colin Campbell. It was the first time in my life anyone had ever argued for eating carbohydrate-rich foods for health and longevity. Prior to this, I had always been told that low-carb diets were the way, the truth and the life, but mostly, of course, for weight-loss purposes.

To say the least, it was a mind-blowing, life-altering moment for me at the time. Here were medical professionals not only giving me permission to eat my biggest fear food, but also encouraging it. Healing my relationship with food might not have happened had I not found advocates for plant-based eating which in a lot of ways is high-carb eating.

Since then, spaghetti and pasta dishes have been a staple in my life, and I am so grateful because, hello, #carbsarelife. In this chapter, you will find some of my absolute favorite recipes for all things noodles that range from more traditional to creative combinations of ingredients and flavors. Some of my favorites include Mushroom Magic (page 89), Al Fresco Pasta (page 90), Sweet Potato Mango-a-Go-Go (page 93) and Nacho Libre Mac & Cheese (page 82).

Nacho Libre Mac & Cheese

What would a cookbook be without a comforting mac & cheese recipe? Incomplete, that's what!
I love the simplicity of this recipe and how much of a crowd-pleaser it is. The creamy nacho cheese sauce
is finger-licking good and goes so well with the crunchy veggie mixture and noodles. Kids and
adults alike will enjoy this one!

SERVES 4

CASHEW NACHO CHEESE

1½ cups (210 g) raw cashews, soaked in very hot water for 12 minutes (see Notes)

½ cup (120 ml) water

1 tbsp (8 g) nutritional yeast

3 tbsp (45 ml) fresh lemon juice

3 tbsp (45 ml) hot sauce of choice; I prefer Cholula

Salt and freshly ground black pepper

PASTA

1 lb (455 g) dried pasta shells

VEGGIES

1 tbsp (14 g) coconut oil

1 medium-sized yellow onion, diced

6 cloves garlic, minced

Salt and freshly ground black pepper

1 red bell pepper, seeded and chopped into bite-size pieces

4 cups (268 g) chopped kale leaves

3 tbsp (45 ml) fresh lemon juice (optional)

Make the nacho cheese: Drain and rinse the cashews, then place in a high-speed blender. Add the fresh water, nutritional yeast, lemon juice, hot sauce and salt and black pepper to taste. Blend on high speed until smooth. Set aside.

Make the pasta: Bring a large pot of salted water to a boil. Add the pasta shells and cook according to the package instructions. Drain and set aside.

While the pasta cooks, make the veggies: In a large skillet, heat the coconut oil over medium-high heat. Once hot, add the onion and cook for 5 minutes, stirring occasionally. Add the garlic, season with salt and black pepper and mix well for 30 seconds. Add the bell pepper and kale. Cook for 10 to 12 minutes, or until the kale is wilted and bell pepper is soft. Add the lemon juice if using, and season with more salt and black pepper to taste.

In a large bowl, combine the pasta, nacho cheese and veggies, then mix well. Divide equally among 4 serving bowls and serve immediately.

Notes: *You can substitute raw sunflower seeds if you want a nut-free version.*

If you do not have a high-speed blender, soak your cashews (or sunflower seeds) for an hour or overnight, to protect your blender.

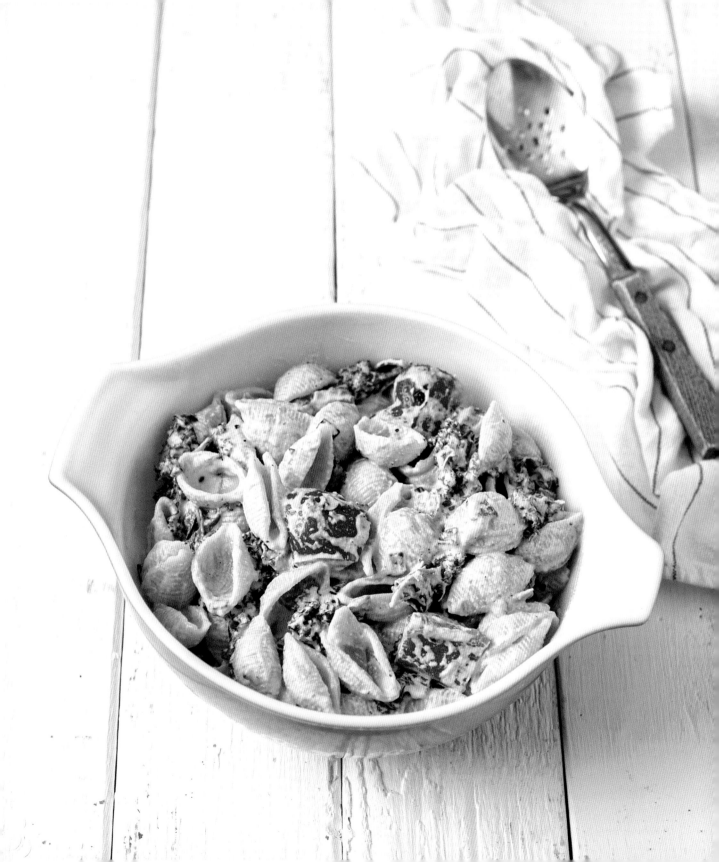

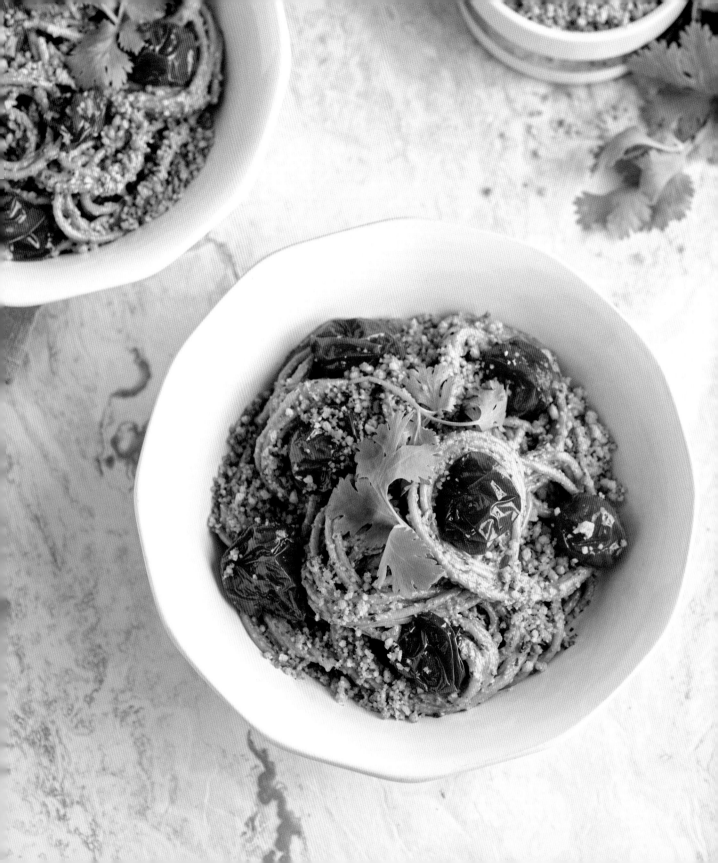

South of the Border Pasta

Without it being the original plan, I married two of my favorite cuisines, Italian and Mexican, and they made this beautiful food baby. The spicy jalapeño and avocado pesto sauce pops on the roasted tomatoes and coats the noodles perfectly. It's topped with a crunchy, cheezy walnut Parmesan topping that absolutely sends this over the top!

SERVES 4

PESTO & WALNUT PARMESAN

1½ cups (150 g) walnuts

½ cup (64 g) nutritional yeast

3 cloves garlic

½ tsp salt, plus more if needed

1 ripe avocado

1½ cups (60 g) chopped cilantro leaves and stems

¼ cup (60 ml) fresh lemon juice

1 jalapeño pepper, chopped

½ cup (120 ml) olive oil

PASTA

1 lb (455 g) whole wheat spaghetti noodles

2 cups (300 g) cherry tomatoes

1 tbsp (15 ml) avocado oil

Salt and freshly ground black pepper

GARNISHES

Fresh cilantro

Preheat the oven to 375°F (190°C) and bring a large pot of salted water to a boil.

Make the pesto: In a food processor fitted with an S blade, combine the walnuts, nutritional yeast, garlic and salt. Pulse in 10-second bursts, 3 times, or until the mixture is reduced to a crumb. Transfer half of the mixture to a small bowl and reserve it to use for the walnut Parmesan. To the remainder in the processor, add the avocado, cilantro, lemon juice and jalapeño. Pulse in 5-second bursts, 4 times, then with the processor on low speed, slowly drizzle in the olive oil through the center of the lid. Taste and add more salt to taste, if desired. Set aside.

Make the pasta: Add the spaghetti to the salted boiling water and cook according to the package instructions. Drain and transfer to a serving bowl.

Lay out the tomatoes on a baking sheet and evenly coat with the avocado oil. Season with salt and pepper. Roast in the oven for 12 minutes, tossing them halfway through the roasting time. Transfer to a plate and set aside.

Make the walnut Parmesan: Carefully, without burning yourself, wipe down the baking sheet with a paper towel to remove any oil. Add the reserved walnut mixture. Roast in the oven for 4 minutes, or until toasted. Keep an eye on it to make sure it doesn't burn.

Add the pesto to the bowl of spaghetti and stir well to evenly coat the noodles. Divide equally among 4 serving bowls, divide the tomatoes among the bowls and sprinkle each bowl generously with the walnut Parmesan. Garnish with fresh cilantro and serve immediately.

"Cheezy" Butternut & Pesto Pasta

The veggie-spiralized-into-noodle movement is clearly something I have gotten behind. Not because I am trying to avoid carbs or gluten, but because it's just so fun to eat all these veggies in the shape of noodles, right? This combination might seem a little bizarre at first, but it works. The sweet butternut squash pairs beautifully with the herbaceous basil pesto and it's rounded out with the creamy cashew cheese. It's simple, yet so good! I am sure you will love it.

SERVES 2

CASHEW CHEESE SAUCE

1 cup (140 g) raw cashews, soaked in very hot water for 12 minutes (see Note)

⅔ cup (160 ml) water

2 cloves garlic

¼ tsp garlic powder

1 tbsp (8 g) nutritional yeast

2 tbsp (30 ml) fresh lemon juice

Salt

PASTA

1 tbsp (14 g) coconut oil

8 cups (600 g) spiralized butternut squash noodles

½ cup (120 ml) water

Salt and freshly ground black pepper

PESTO

1 prepared recipe Basil Pesto (page 135)

Make the cheese sauce: Drain and rinse the cashews and place them in a high-speed blender. Add the ⅔ cup (160 ml) of fresh water, garlic cloves, garlic powder, nutritional yeast, lemon juice and salt to taste. Blend on high speed until smooth. Taste and see whether you want to add any more of the seasonings. Set aside.

Make the pasta: In a large, lidded skillet, heat the coconut oil over medium heat. Once hot, add the butternut squash noodles and cook for 10 minutes, stirring often. Add the water, cover and lower the heat to medium-low. Let simmer, tossing every 2 minutes, for 6 to 10 minutes, or until the liquid is absorbed.

Remove the lid and sauté, tossing frequently, for another 3 to 5 minutes, or until cooked through and soft to the bite. Season with salt and pepper to taste. Turn off the heat and add the cheese sauce. Mix well to evenly coat the noodles.

Divide the noodles equally among 2 serving bowls and top each bowl with a generous spoonful of basil pesto. Serve immediately.

Note: If you do not have a high-speed blender, soak your cashews for an hour or overnight, to protect your blender.

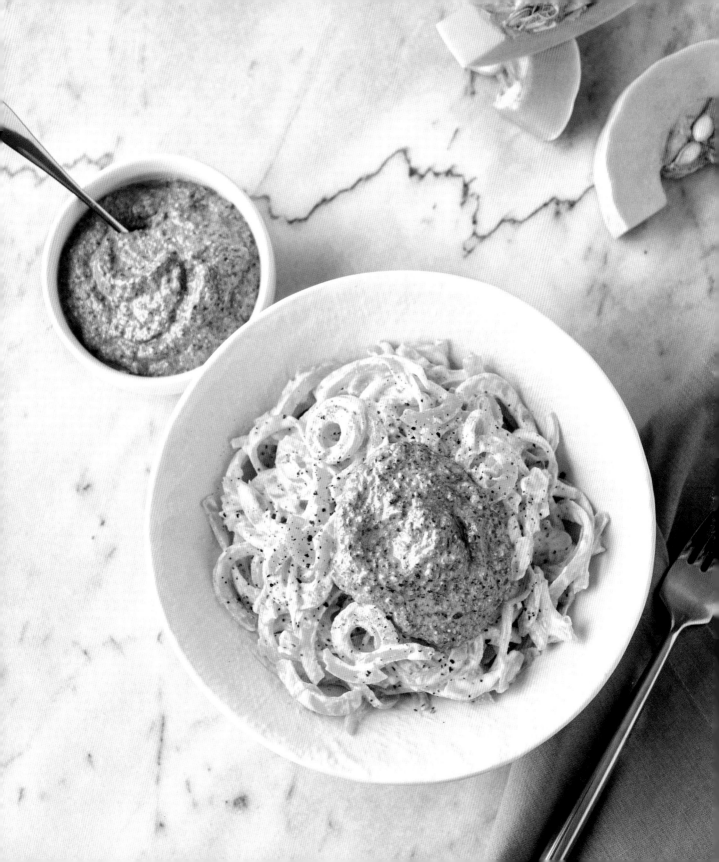

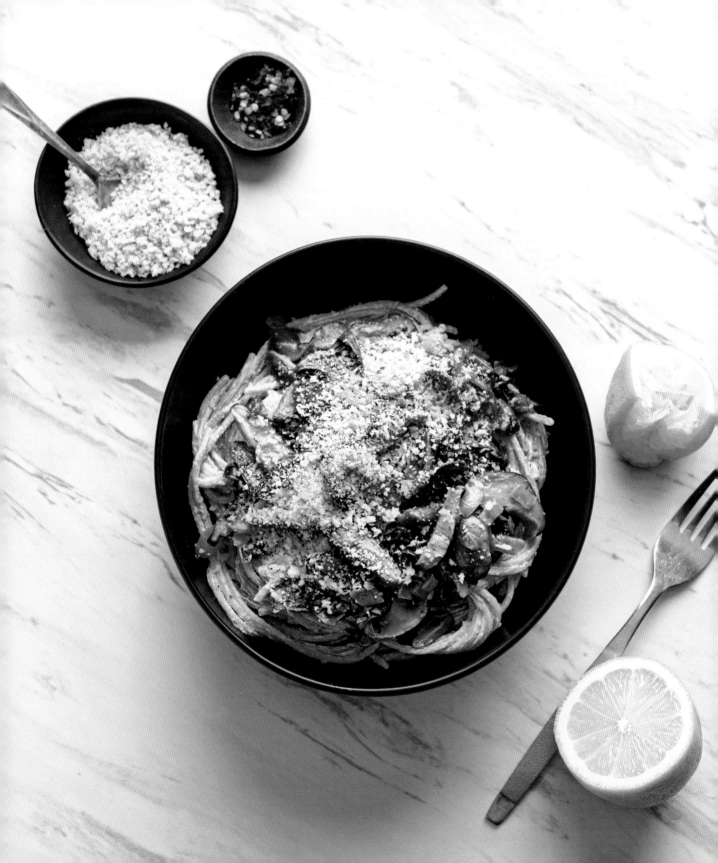

Mushroom Magic

Pasta is always on high rotation at my place, so I often put on my creative kitchen witch hat and fuse together different cuisines to keep things fresh and interesting. This one mixes Italian-style spaghetti with a light Asian twist that is comforting and seriously flavorful. The rich cashew Alfredo sauce beautifully coats the noodles and the silky mushrooms and spinach add some texture and necessary complexity. This is an easy, quick, decadent meal that is a so easy to fall in love with!

SERVES 4

SAUCE

1 cup (140 g) raw cashews, soaked in very hot water for 12 minutes (see Note)

⅓ cup (80 ml) water

1 clove garlic

1 tbsp (15 ml) tamari or soy sauce

1 tbsp (15 ml) apple cider vinegar

Juice of ½ to 1 lemon

2 to 3 tsp (6 to 8 g) nutritional yeast

½ tsp garlic powder

Crushed red pepper flakes

Freshly ground black pepper

PASTA

1 lb (455 g) whole wheat spaghetti noodles

1 to 2 tsp (5 to 10 ml) olive oil

Salt

VEGGIES

1 tbsp (14 g) coconut oil

1 medium-sized onion, diced

4 cups (280 g) sliced cremini mushrooms

2 cups (134 g) sliced shiitake mushrooms

4 cloves garlic, minced

½ tsp garlic powder

1 tbsp (15 ml) tamari or soy sauce

Big pinch of red pepper flakes

3 to 4 handfuls of spinach or chopped kale

GARNISHES

Fresh lemon juice

Crushed red pepper flakes (optional)

Vegan panko bread crumbs (optional)

Nutritional yeast or store-bought vegan Parmesan cheese (optional)

Make the sauce: Drain and rinse the cashews, then place in a high-speed blender. Add the fresh water, garlic clove, tamari, vinegar, lemon juice, nutritional yeast, garlic powder, red pepper flakes and black pepper and blend on high speed until smooth. Taste and see if you want to add any more of the seasonings. Set aside.

Make the pasta: Bring a large pot of salted water to a boil, then cook the spaghetti according to the package directions. Drain the noodles, reserving ⅓ cup (80 ml) of the starchy cooking water. In a large bowl, combine the noodles and reserved starchy water with the olive oil and salt to taste. Toss the noodles so they do not stick together. Set aside.

Make the veggies: Heat the coconut oil in a large skillet over medium heat. Once hot, add the onion and sauté for 3 to 5 minutes. Add the mushrooms and cook down for 5 to 6 minutes. Once their liquid has released, add the minced garlic, garlic powder, tamari and red pepper flakes and cook, stirring, for 3 to 4 minutes. Lower the heat to low, toss in the spinach and cook, stirring, to wilt, 1 to 2 minutes.

Add the sauce to the bowl of noodles and mix well to evenly coat. Divide the noodles equally among 4 serving bowls, then divide the mushroom mixture among the bowls. Add a squeeze of lemon juice plus red pepper flakes, panko and/or nutritional yeast (if using). Serve immediately.

Note: If you do not have a high-speed blender, soak your cashews for an hour or overnight, to protect your blender.

Al Fresco Pasta

I didn't think it was possible for traditional spaghetti to get better, but it turns out that, by adding zucchini noodles, it can. I love the additional crunchy element they add, plus getting in extra vegetables is always something my body appreciates. The butter–basil sauce is rich and pungent in flavor and fragrance; you can't help but be a little intoxicated by it! The roasted tomatoes, pine nuts and nutritional yeast make this a complete meal that is perfect for some al fresco dining!

SERVES 4

ROASTED TOMATOES

2 cups (300 g) cherry tomatoes

1 tbsp (15 ml) avocado oil

Salt and freshly ground black pepper

BUTTER–BASIL SAUCE

1 cup (225 g) vegan butter

¼ cup (60 ml) olive oil

10 cloves garlic, minced

⅓ cup (17 g) tightly packed chopped fresh basil

¼ cup (60 ml) fresh lemon juice

Salt and freshly ground black pepper

VEGGIES & PASTA

4 medium-sized zucchini, spiralized into noodles

1 lb (455 g) spaghetti noodles

1 (15-oz [425-g]) can garbanzo beans, drained and rinsed

GARNISHES

Pine nuts

Nutritional yeast

Preheat the oven to 350°F (180°C).

Make the tomatoes: In a bowl, toss the tomatoes with the avocado oil and salt and pepper to taste. Lay out in a single layer on a baking sheet and roast in the oven for 20 to 25 minutes. Remove from the oven and set aside.

Make the sauce: In a large saucepan, melt the butter over medium-low heat. Once hot, add the olive oil, garlic, basil, lemon juice and salt and pepper to taste. Cook, stirring occasionally, for 7 to 10 minutes.

Add the zucchini noodles to the sauce, cover and cook, stirring occasionally, for another 10 minutes, or until the noodles are softened. Set aside.

Bring a large pot of water to a boil and cook the spaghetti according to the package instructions.

Rinse and drain the spaghetti, transfer to a large bowl and add the zucchini noodle mixture, garbanzo beans and tomatoes. Divide equally among 4 serving bowls and top with pine nuts and nutritional yeast.

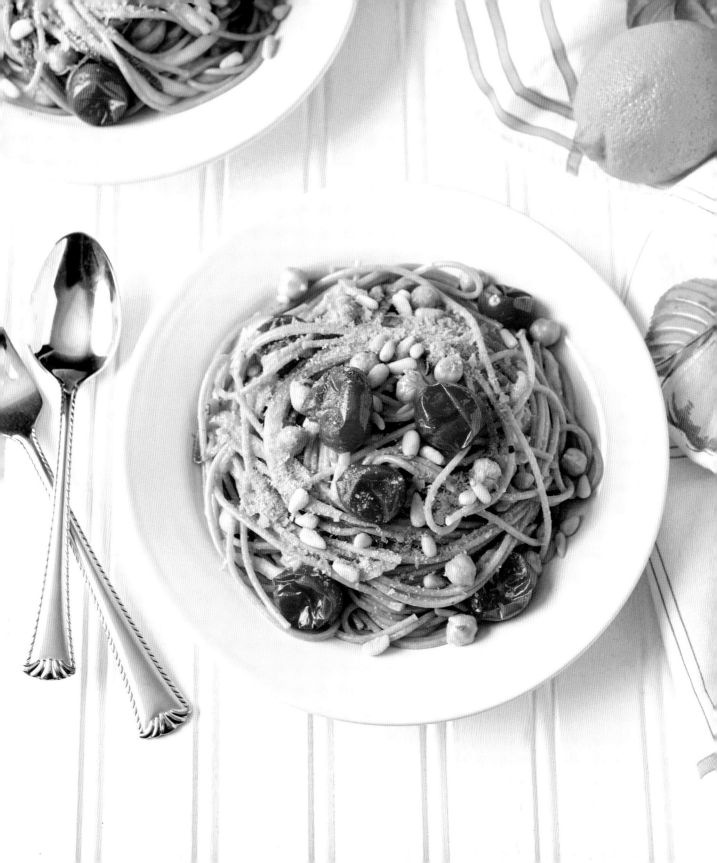

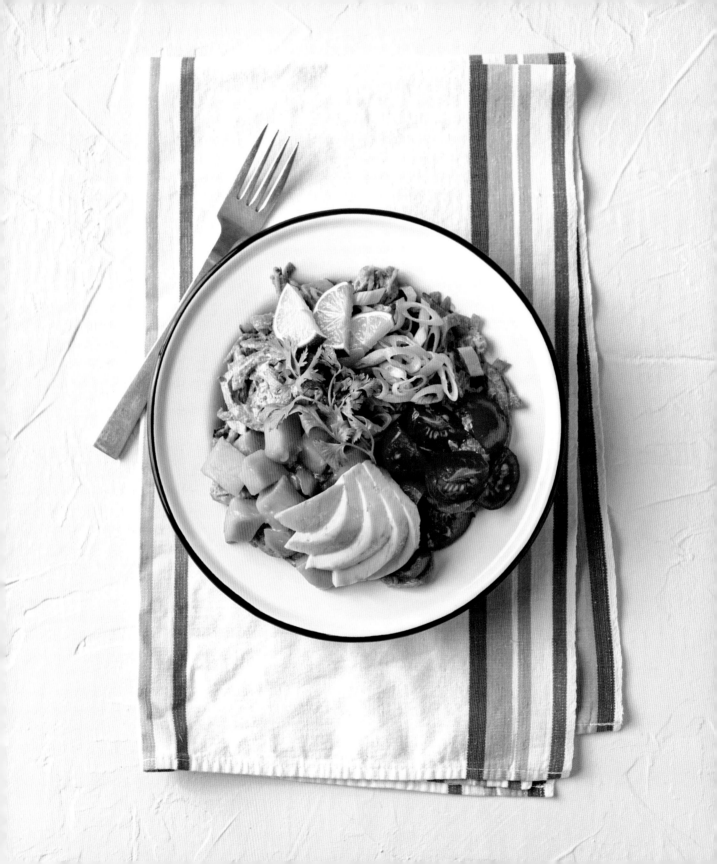

Sweet Potato Mango-a-Go-Go

When my boyfriend first tried this recipe, he said that if Thanksgiving were in the Bahamas, this is how they'd do the sweet potatoes. I can't help but find that shockingly accurate! The color alone makes it feel extra tropical. But the mango really gives it that feel and its refreshing sweetness is a must with the grounding sweet potato noodles, thick and creamy sauce and avocado. Needless to say, this is such a fun dish and I hope you enjoy it.

SERVES 4

CASHEW NACHO CHEESE

1½ cups (210 g) raw cashews, soaked in very hot water for 12 minutes (see Note)

½ cup (120 ml) water

1 tbsp (8 g) nutritional yeast

2 tbsp (30 ml) fresh lemon juice

3 tbsp (45 ml) hot sauce of choice; I prefer Cholula

Salt and freshly ground black pepper

PASTA

⅓ cup (75 g) coconut oil, divided

14 cups (1.1 kg) spiralized sweet potato noodles (from 3 to 4 large sweet potatoes)

¾ cup (175 ml) water, divided

1 to 2 tsp (3 to 6 g) garlic powder

1 to 2 tsp (2 to 5 g) chili powder

1 tsp salt

Freshly ground black pepper

1 large ripe mango, peeled, pitted and cut into ½" (1.2-cm) cubes

2 cups (300 g) chopped cherry tomatoes

1 large ripe avocado, sliced

GARNISHES

Fresh cilantro

Green onion

Crushed red pepper flakes

Red onion

Lime wedges

Make the nacho cheese: Drain and rinse the cashews, then place in a high-speed blender. Add the fresh water, nutritional yeast, lemon juice, hot sauce and salt and pepper to taste. Blend on high speed until smooth. Set aside.

Make the pasta: To ensure even cooking, cook the sweet potato noodles in 3 batches. In a large, lidded skillet, melt 2 tablespoons (28 g) of the coconut oil over medium heat and add a third of the sweet potato noodles. Cook for 5 minutes, stirring occasionally. Then add ¼ cup (60 ml) of the water and cover. Let simmer for 5 minutes, or until all the liquid is absorbed. Remove the lid and cook, stirring occasionally, for another 2 to 3 minutes, or until fully softened. Transfer to a large bowl. Repeat 2 more times to cook the remaining noodles and add them to the bowl. Once they are all cooked, add the garlic powder, chili powder, salt and black pepper to taste and mix well to combine.

Add the sauce and mix well to evenly coat all the noodles. Add half of the mango and tomatoes and mix well. Divide equally among 4 serving bowls and divide the remaining mango and tomatoes among the bowls. Top each bowl with the avocado slices. Garnish with the cilantro, green onion, red pepper flakes, red onion and lime wedges and dig in!

Note: *If you do not have a high-speed blender, soak your cashews for an hour or overnight, to protect your blender.*

Kale 'em with Kindness

*A fireplace, people you love, a glass of red wine and this pasta—pure cozy perfection.
The sweetness of the butternut squash and cranberries is balanced out by the smoke-flavored onions
and bitter kale, then coated with the tangy yet creamy cashew ricotta. It is seriously a recipe from above.
It is easy to make, but has so much complexity in taste and texture!*

--------- SERVES 4 ---------

CASHEW RICOTTA

1½ cups (210 g) raw cashews, soaked in very hot water for 12 minutes (see Note)

½ cup (120 ml) water

¼ cup (60 ml) fresh lemon juice

2 cloves garlic

1 tbsp (8 g) nutritional yeast

Salt and freshly ground black pepper

PASTA

1 lb (455 g) whole wheat spaghetti noodles

¼ cup (60 ml) olive oil

2 tbsp (30 ml) fresh lemon juice

Salt

VEGGIES & CRANBERRIES

4 cups (560 g) cubed butternut squash (½" [1.2-cm] cubes)

¼ cup (55 g) coconut oil, divided

½ tsp garlic powder

Salt

1 medium-sized onion, sliced thinly into half-moons

1 tbsp (15 ml) liquid smoke, plus more to taste

5 cups (335 g) chopped kale

Freshly ground black pepper

½ cup (60 g) dried cranberries

Make the cashew ricotta: Drain and rinse the cashews, then place in a high-speed blender. Add the fresh water, lemon juice, garlic, nutritional yeast, salt and pepper. Blend on high speed until smooth, stopping to scrape down the sides, if necessary.

Make the pasta: Bring a large pot of salted water to a boil. Cook the spaghetti according to the package directions. Drain the noodles, reserving ⅓ cup (80 ml) of the starchy cooking water. In a large bowl, combine the spaghetti and reserved starchy water with the olive oil and lemon juice. Season generously with salt. Toss the noodles so they do not stick together. Set aside.

Meanwhile, preheat the oven to 450°F (230°C).

Make the veggies: In a bowl, toss the butternut squash in 2 tablespoons (28 g) of the coconut oil, add the garlic powder, season with salt and lay out in a single layer on a baking sheet. Roast in the oven for 12 to 14 minutes, or until fork tender. Remove from the oven and set aside.

In a large skillet, heat the remaining 2 tablespoons (28 g) of the coconut oil over medium heat. Once hot, add the onion and lower the heat to medium-low. Cook, stirring often, for 12 minutes. Add the liquid smoke and cook, stirring, for another 2 minutes. Add the kale and sauté until wilted. Season generously with salt and pepper.

Add the butternut squash, veggie mixture, cashew ricotta and dried cranberries to the bowl of pasta. Mix well to evenly coat, then divide equally among 4 serving bowls.

Note: *If you do not have a high-speed blender, soak your cashews for an hour or overnight, to protect your blender.*

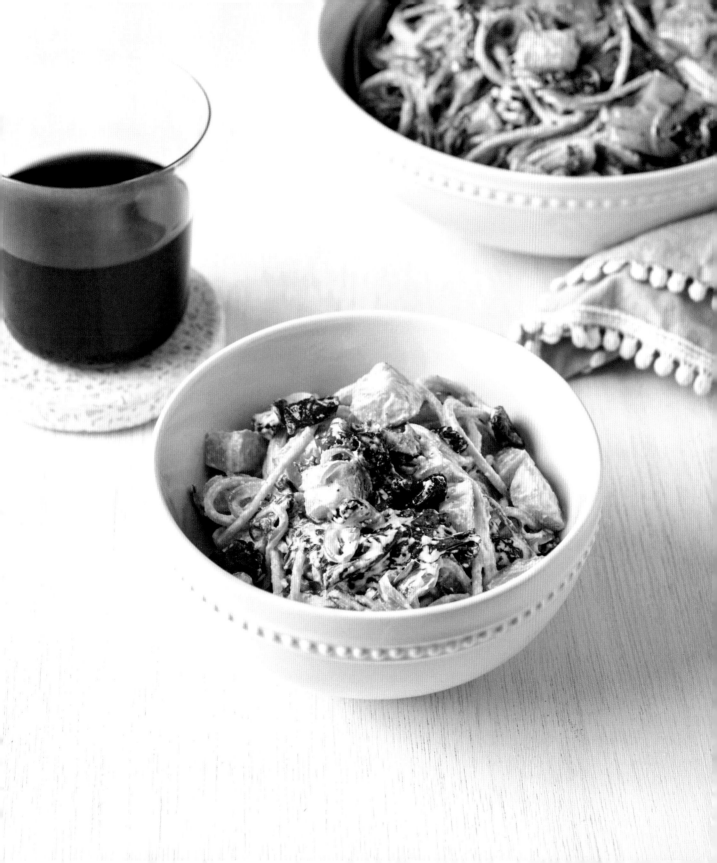

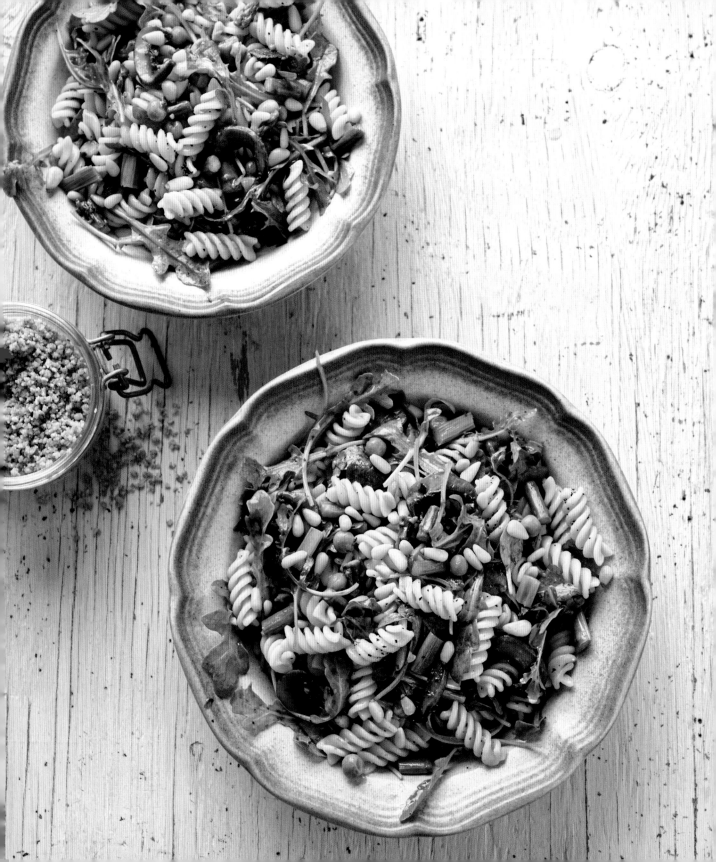

The Lemony Veg Pasta

I love this easy, flavorful and colorful pasta salad. It was actually a really popular "grab 'n' go" item at my old café, Superette, and I am so happy that a piece of that is living on in this book. The acidic and bright lemon juice and zest totally shine next to the peppery arugula and crunchy vegetables. The savory mushrooms balance out the flavor and the pasta noodles become the perfect vehicle for each delicious bite!

SERVES 4

PASTA SALAD

1 tbsp (14 g) coconut oil

5 cloves garlic, minced

2 cups (140 g) thinly sliced cremini mushrooms

Salt and freshly ground black pepper

2 cups (168 g) chopped asparagus spears (½" [1.2-cm] pieces)

½ cup (75 g) sweet peas

1 lb (455 g) fusilli pasta

1 tbsp (15 ml) olive oil

4 cups (88 g) tightly packed arugula

2 tsp (2 g) crushed red pepper flakes

DRESSING

Zest and juice of 3 medium-sized lemons

⅔ cup (160 ml) olive oil

2 tsp (6 g) garlic powder

Salt and freshly ground black pepper

GARNISHES

Walnut Parmesan (page 85; alternatively prepare with cashews)

Pine nuts or chopped almonds

Make the salad: In a large skillet over medium heat, melt the coconut oil. Once hot, add the garlic and mushrooms. Cook stirring every 2 to 3 minutes, for 6 to 8 minutes, or until the mushrooms have released their liquid, then season with salt and black pepper to taste. Add the asparagus and cook, stirring occasionally, for 10 to 12 minutes, or until the mushrooms are cooked through and the asparagus are cooked but still crunchy. If the peas are frozen, defrost them with hot water and then drain. Transfer the cooked veggies and peas to a large bowl. Set aside.

Bring a large pot of salted water to a boil. Cook the fusilli according to the package instructions. Drain, then transfer the noodles to the bowl of veggies. Add the olive oil and toss to coat so the pasta doesn't stick. Season with salt and black pepper to taste. Set aside to cool for 5 to 10 minutes, then add the arugula and red pepper flakes.

Make the dressing: In a small bowl, whisk together the lemon zest and juice, olive oil, garlic powder, salt and black pepper. Pour over the pasta salad, mix well and serve immediately.

If desired, top with walnut Parmesan and pine nuts.

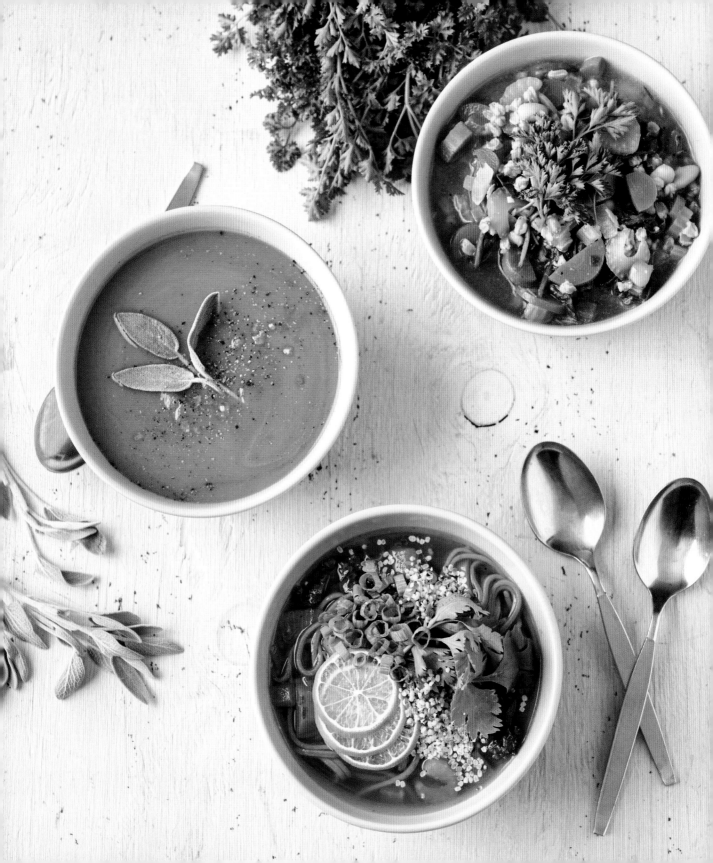

Easy Plant-Powered Soups

I've always loved soup. When I was younger, I mostly opted for canned varieties, and while I still appreciate the convenience factor, I find homemade soups to be not too much additional effort but so high on the ROI (return on investment) that it's totally worth it.

In this chapter, you will find some of the simplest yet most surprisingly flavorful soups that have been enjoyed by many before making their way into this book. I've prepared several of these recipes at women's retreats, so I know that some just might cause a dance party in your mouth! Plus they are loaded with nutrient-rich veggies that your body will thank you for. I just love to cozy up on the couch with a comforting bowl of soup!

Most of these soups can be prepared in advance for meal prep, including the Creamy Broccoli Soup (page 103), Pea & Corn Chowder (page 104), Creamy Cauliflower & Leek Soup (page 107), Farro & Vegetable Soup (page 108) and Simple Sage–Butternut Squash Soup (page 111). If making ahead, mix everything together as directed and store in an airtight container in the fridge for up to a week or for one month in the freezer.

Vibrant Turmeric Vegetable Noodle Soup

This soup literally brings me a sense of happiness. Maybe it's the vibrant color, the healing nature of ginger and turmeric or the fact that the child in me that likes to slurp soup gets to come out. Whatever it is, it works.

It's a hearty, comforting recipe with a good broth-to-noodle-to-vegetable ratio that I always aim for when creating a soup of this kind. That makes it more of a complete meal than a side dish! Not only is it bright and flavorful, but it's loaded with ingredients that are good for your body and soul, plus nutrients that you can all-around enjoy eating.

SERVES 4

2 tbsp (28 g) coconut oil

1 medium-sized white or yellow onion, diced

4 medium-sized carrots, peeled and chopped into half-moons

2 to 3 ribs celery, chopped in half-moons

Salt and freshly ground black pepper

5 cloves garlic, minced

1 (1" [2.5-cm]) knob fresh ginger, grated (preferred) or minced

1 tbsp (7 g) ground turmeric

1½ tsp (5 g) garlic powder

1 to 2 tsp (1 to 2 g) crushed red pepper flakes

3 quarts (2.8 L) vegetable broth

3 green onions, light and dark green parts, sliced

2 cups (134 g) loosely packed chopped curly kale

Juice of 1 lime

1 tbsp (15 ml) pure maple syrup or honey (optional, but rounds out the flavors)

6 oz (170 g) dried soba noodles

GARNISHES

Fresh cilantro

Green onion

Lime wedges

Crushed red pepper flakes

Hemp seeds

In a large soup pot, melt the coconut oil over medium heat. Once hot, add the onion, carrots and celery. Sauté the veggies for 6 to 7 minutes, or until they're lightly softened and the onion is translucent. Season generously with a pinch of salt and black pepper and stir.

Add the garlic cloves and ginger and cook, stirring well, for 30 seconds. Add the turmeric, garlic powder and red pepper flakes and mix well to coat all the vegetables. Add the vegetable broth and the green onions. Taste and see whether you want to adjust any of the seasonings.

Bring to a boil, then lower the heat to a simmer and cook for 10 to 12 minutes to let the flavors blend. Add the kale, lime juice and maple syrup (if using). Stir well and then turn off the heat.

While the soup is simmering, prepare the noodles in a separate pot according to the package instructions.

Add the cooked noodles to the soup before serving. If you'd like, top with fresh cilantro, green onion, lime wedges, red pepper flakes and hemp seeds.

This soup is best enjoyed fresh. It doesn't keep especially well, since the noodles tend to soak up more liquid and get soggy.

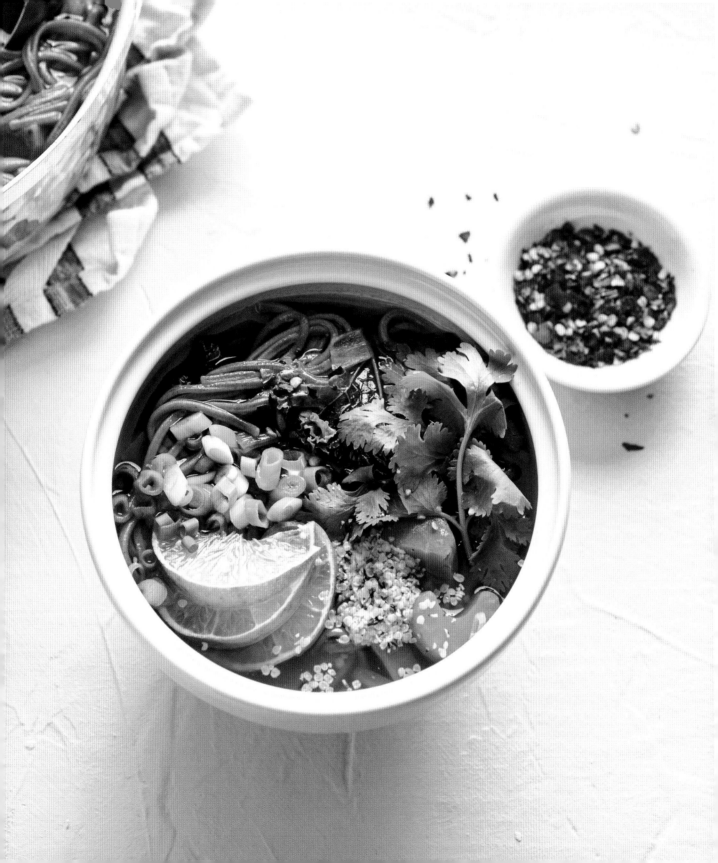

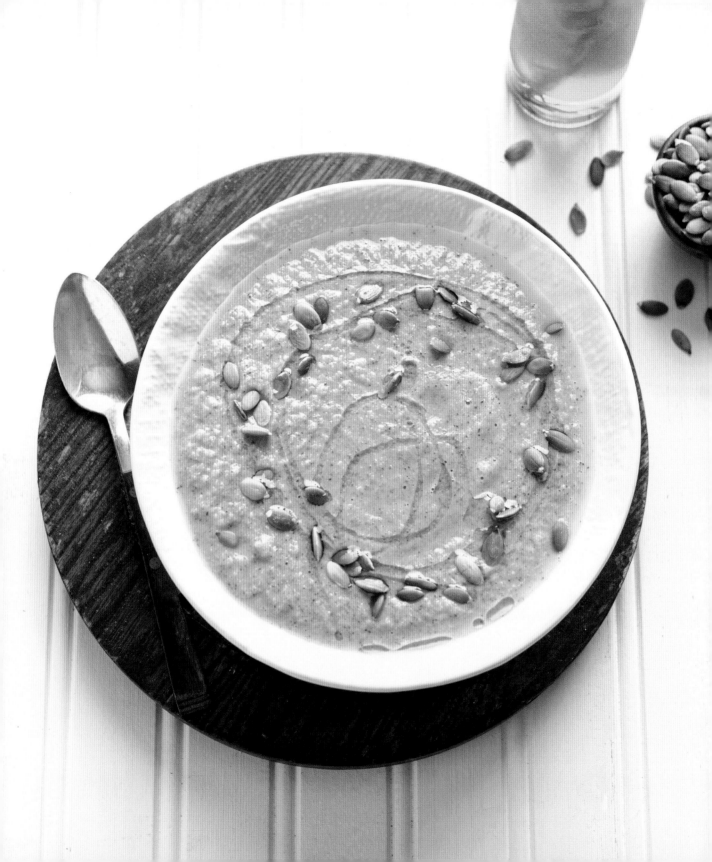

Creamy Broccoli Soup

Since I was a kid, I have loved broccoli soup of pretty much any kind and this one is no exception. Not only is it incredibly easy to make, but the flavor is so well rounded. The cumin and lemon really add something special, while the garbanzo beans provide a creamy texture. You'll be surprised how delicious it is with so few ingredients. Serve it up with some crusty bread and you'll have yourself an easy, healthy meal.

SERVES 4

1 tbsp (14 g) coconut oil

1 large yellow onion, diced

Salt and freshly ground black pepper

5 cloves garlic, minced

24 oz (680 g) broccoli florets

1 tsp garlic powder

1 heaping tbsp (8 g) ground cumin

5 cups (1.2 L) vegetable broth

2 tbsp (30 ml) fresh lemon juice

1 (15-oz [425-g]) can garbanzo beans (chickpeas), drained, rinsed and skins removed (see Note)

TO SERVE

4 slices crusty vegan bread

Pepitas

Drizzle of olive oil

In a large soup pot, heat the coconut oil over medium heat. Once hot, add the onion and season with salt and pepper to taste. Sauté for 5 minutes, stirring occasionally.

Add the minced garlic, broccoli florets, garlic powder, cumin and salt to taste. Cook, stirring occasionally, for another 2 to 3 minutes, then add the vegetable broth and bring to a boil. Cover, lower the heat to a simmer and cook for 10 minutes, or until the broccoli is softened. Add the lemon juice and garbanzo beans and mix well.

Working in batches, transfer to a blender and puree until very smooth. Taste to see whether you want to add any more vegetable broth, salt or spices, and add black pepper to taste. Serve immediately with a slice of bread, pepitas and a drizzle of olive oil on top of the soup.

Note: *To remove the skins from the chickpeas, lay out a clean dish towel on the counter. Place half of the beans in the center of the towel and gently fold over all four sides to enclose the beans. Then using your hands, gently apply pressure to the beans and move your hands in a circular motion for 15 to 30 seconds to loosen the skins. Unwrap the towel and discard the skins. There may be some that you will need to remove by hand. To do so, pinch the bean between 2 to 3 fingers to release the skin and discard. Repeat for the remaining beans. This makes the soup extra creamy and is absolutely worth the extra effort!*

Pea & Corn Chowder

One of my favorite things to do is chef at women's retreats. Because of the large group of people, I have to get creative in the kitchen, coming up with recipes that meet everyone's dietary requirements. This is a fun take on a classic chowder that uses cauliflower instead of potatoes to make it nightshade-free, and it is delicious. After partial blending it has a lovely thick texture, and the corn and peas add a beautiful sweetness that is tied together perfectly with the thyme and rosemary. You will love this!

SERVES 4

1 tbsp (14 g) coconut oil

1 large yellow onion

Salt and freshly ground black pepper

4 cloves garlic, minced

1 large head cauliflower, chopped into small pieces (see Note)

2 tbsp (5 g) fresh thyme leaves

1 tbsp (2 g) chopped fresh rosemary

4 cups (946 ml) vegetable broth

1 lb (455 g) frozen sweet peas

1 lb (455 g) frozen corn kernels

In a large soup pot, melt the coconut oil over medium heat. Once hot, add the onion and season with salt and pepper. Sauté for 5 minutes, then add the garlic, cauliflower, thyme and rosemary. Season again with salt and pepper to taste and mix well. Cook for 7 minutes, stirring occasionally.

Add the vegetable broth and bring to a boil, then add the peas and corn. Lower the heat to a simmer and cook, stirring, for another 3 to 5 minutes. Transfer half of the mixture to a high-speed blender and puree until smooth.

Transfer the puree back to the soup pot and stir to combine. Taste the soup and see whether you would like to add any more salt and pepper, then serve.

Note: *Chop the florets into small pieces, only a little bigger than the size of the peas and corn.*

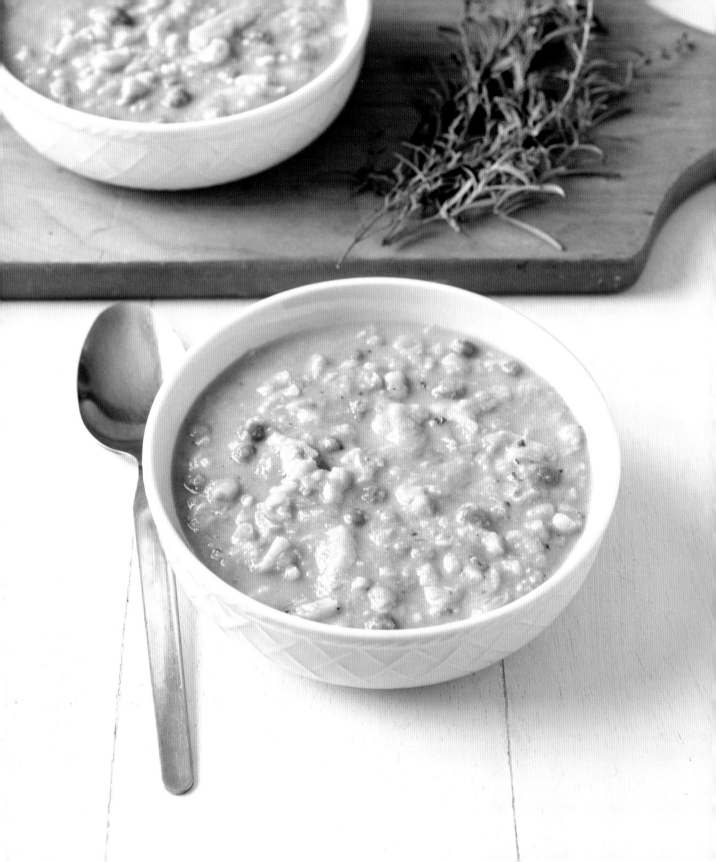

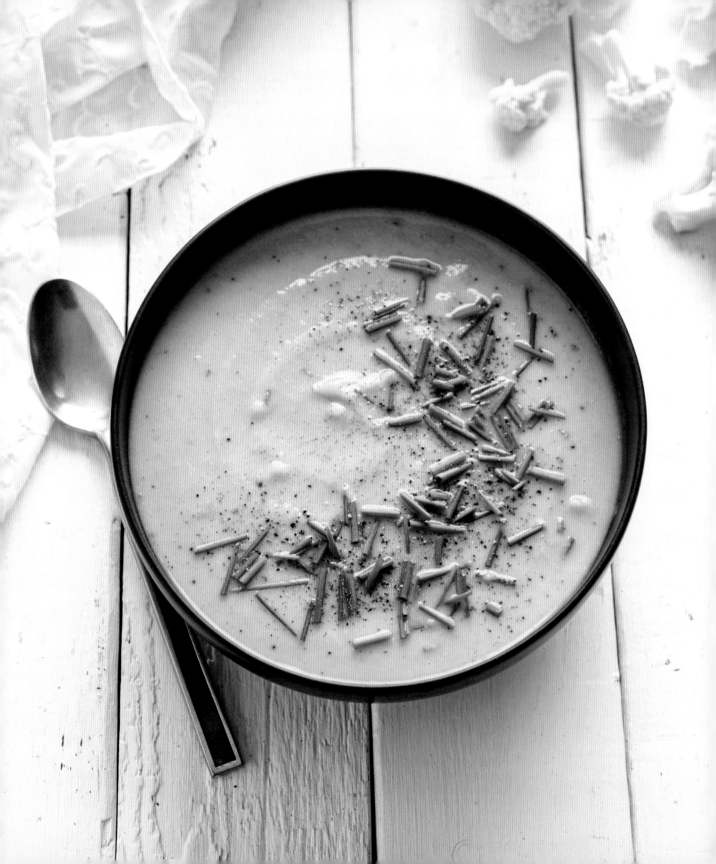

Creamy Cauliflower & Leek Soup

Some might think that this soup is a crime against the potato, so please know my intention with it was not to make a "low-carb" version that was better for your waistline. I am not into that diet culture hoopla. As I mentioned in the previous recipe, nightshades are often a food allergen I must work around when cooking for large groups of people, so that is how this delicious soup was born.

The creamy cauliflower is just as comforting as traditional potato and pairs perfectly with leeks. The smell while cooking is delightfully pungent, and once blended, the soup becomes a flavor and texture powerhouse. It's such a fun, easy and delicious way to get in loads of fibrous vegetables, too.

SERVES 2

2 tbsp (28 g) vegan butter

2 large leeks, white and light green parts only, well rinsed and roughly chopped (about 2½ cups [260 g])

3 cloves garlic, minced

6 cups (600 g) chopped cauliflower florets (½" [1.2-cm] pieces)

4 cups (946 ml) vegetable broth

1 bay leaf

2 sprigs thyme

1 tsp salt

½ tsp freshly ground black pepper

2 tbsp (6 g) chopped fresh chives, plus more for garnish

In a large soup pot, melt the butter over medium heat. Once hot, add the leeks and garlic and sauté for about 10 minutes, adjusting the heat as necessary so you do not brown them.

Add the cauliflower, vegetable broth, bay leaf, thyme and salt and pepper to the pot and bring to a boil. Cover and lower the heat to a simmer. Cook for 12 to 15 minutes, stirring occasionally to make sure all the cauliflower cooks.

Remove the thyme sprigs and bay leaf. Working in batches, transfer the soup to a high-speed blender to puree. Once everything is pureed, stir in the chives. Serve immediately and garnish with more chives, if desired.

Farro & Vegetable Soup

Pretty much year-round, I can be in the mood for an easy broth-based soup, and this one totally fits the bill. Although it uses simple vegetables, such as carrot, celery and spinach, it feels extra special with the combination of spices, farro and northern beans. Surely, you will love this simple, soothing soup.

SERVES 4

1 tbsp (14 g) coconut oil

1 large onion, chopped

4 ribs celery, thinly sliced

4 carrots, sliced into thin half-moons

Salt and freshly ground black pepper

6 cloves garlic, minced

1 tbsp (7 g) onion powder

1 tbsp (3 g) dried rosemary

1 tsp crushed red pepper flakes

1 cup (200 g) pearled farro (see Note)

8 cups (1.9 L) vegetable broth

1 (15-oz [425 g]) can great northern beans

3 cups (95 g) tightly packed spinach

GARNISH

Fresh parsley

In a large soup pot, melt the coconut oil over medium heat. Once hot, add the onion, celery and carrots. Season generously with salt and black pepper and cook for 3 to 5 minutes, stirring occasionally. Add the garlic, onion powder, rosemary and red pepper flakes and cook, stirring, for 1 minute.

Add the farro and stir to evenly coat. Cook for about 2 minutes, then pour in the vegetable broth and bring to a boil over high heat. Lower the heat to medium and cook, stirring often, until the farro is almost tender, about 3 minutes.

Add the beans and spinach and cook for another 3 to 5 minutes, or until the farro is tender. Add salt and pepper to taste.

Divide the soup equally among 4 serving bowls, garnish with fresh parsley and serve.

Note: *Make sure to buy pearled or quick-cooking farro; otherwise, the cooking time will vary.*

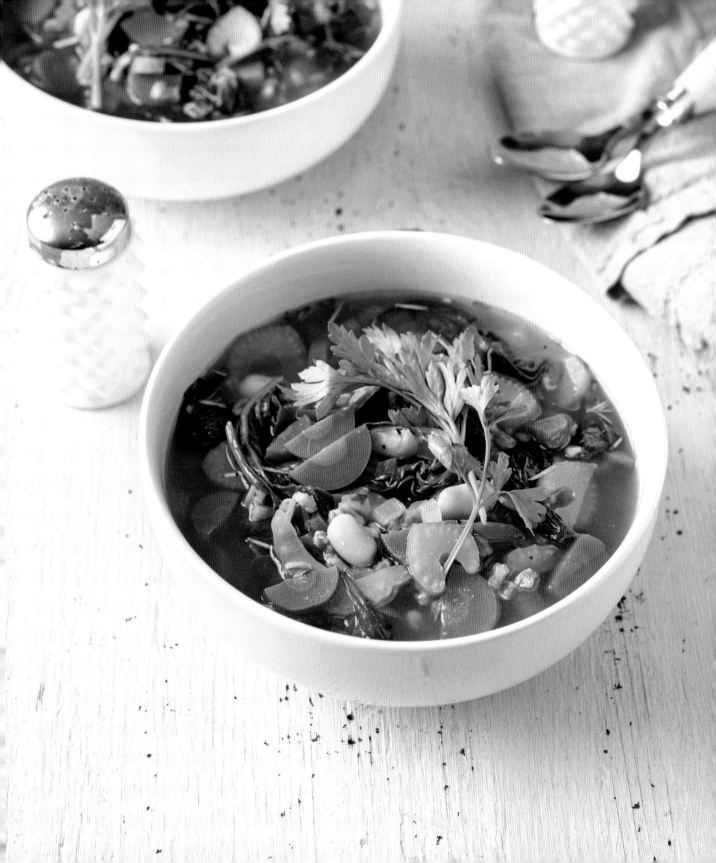

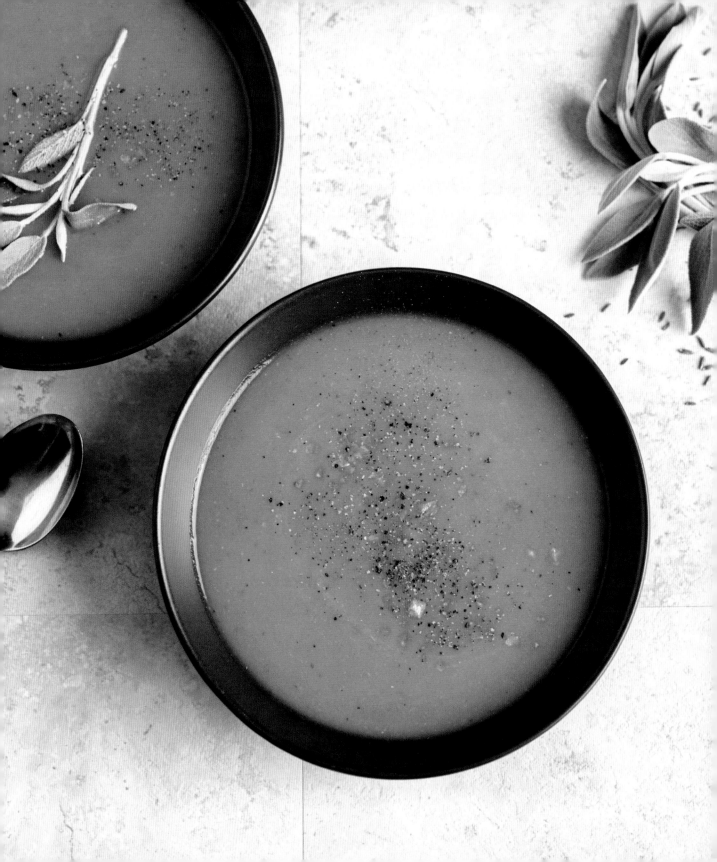

Simple Sage–Butternut Squash Soup

Soups already tend to be on the easier side, in my opinion, since you're mostly combining everything in one pot. This recipe has that going for it (minus the blender action), but it has so much complexity in flavor from such few ingredients that you wouldn't know it otherwise. Sage pairs so beautifully with squash and root vegetables that it is a classic combination, but the addition of cumin and curry powder brings something new to the table. Serve this with some crusty bread and you will be in heaven.

SERVES 4

1 tbsp (14 g) coconut oil

1 medium-sized yellow onion, diced

Pink salt

6 cloves garlic, minced

2 tsp (5 g) curry powder (Indian variety with turmeric)

1 tsp cumin powder

2 tbsp (5 g) chopped fresh sage

Freshly ground black pepper

8 cups (1120 g) cubed butternut squash (1" [2.5-cm] cubes)

4 cups (946 ml) vegetable broth

Juice of 1 lime

In a large soup pot, melt the coconut oil over medium heat. Once hot, add the onion and cook for 3 to 5 minutes. Season with pink salt to taste. Add the garlic, curry powder, cumin and sage and cook, stirring, for 1 minute, then season again with a pinch each of pink salt and pepper. Add the butternut squash and cook for 7 minutes, stirring occasionally. Add the vegetable broth. Bring to a boil, then lower the heat to a simmer and cook, stirring occasionally, for 7 minutes.

Working in batches, transfer the soup to a high-speed blender. Blending on high speed, puree until smooth. Add the lime juice, then season with more salt and pepper to taste.

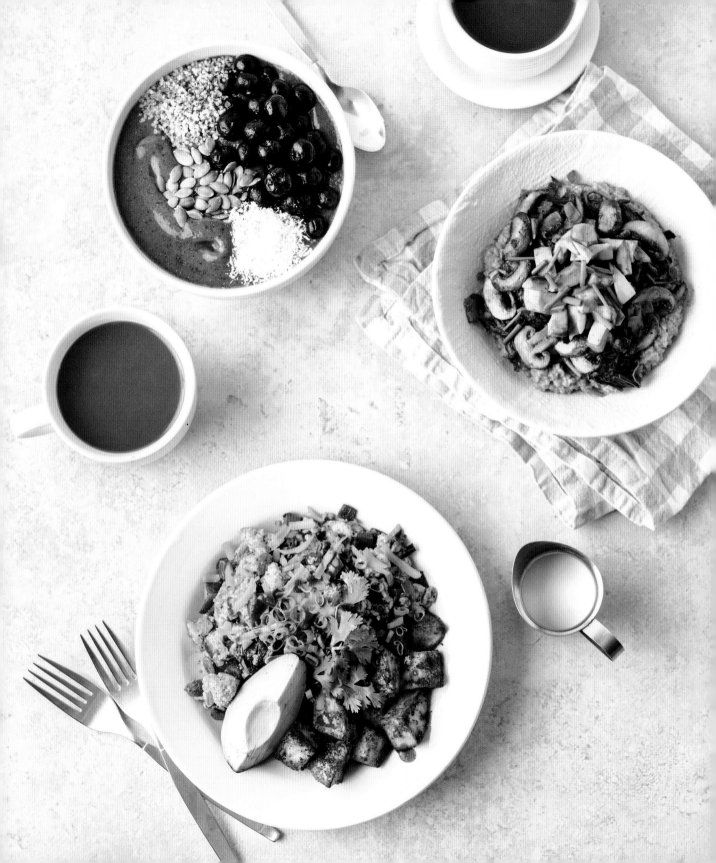

Energizing Breakfast Bowls

They say breakfast is the most important meal of the day, and while I would argue all meals are important, it's never a bad idea to start your day with an energizing breakfast bowl! Whether you are the type who prefers something on the sweeter side (in which case, do not miss out on the Caramelized Banana Smoothie Bowl, page 118), or you lean more toward the savory side of life (be sure to get down with the Savory Mushroom Oatmeal, page 117), you will find a powerful plant-based breakfast to kick-start your day!

Mexi-Cali Tofu Scramble

Without a doubt, I am a surefire savory girl and would take a delicious scramble over pancakes ten out of ten times. After tasting this one, you might see why! It is spiced to perfection and has some crunch from the bell peppers, so the texture is perfect. Topped off with avocado, hot sauce and fresh herbs, this quick, nutritious and filling breakfast will likely be a household favorite!

SERVES 4

POTATOES

4 cups (550 g) cubed russet potato (1" [2.5-cm] cubes)

3 tbsp (45 ml) melted coconut oil

1 tbsp (9 g) garlic powder

2 tsp (5 g) ground cumin

2 tsp (5 g) smoked paprika

Salt and freshly ground black pepper

SCRAMBLE

2 (15.5-oz [439-g]) packages extra-firm tofu, drained and rinsed

2 tbsp (28 g) coconut oil

1 medium-sized red onion, diced

Salt and freshly ground black pepper

1 large red bell pepper, seeded and diced

4 cloves garlic, minced

2 tsp (5 g) smoked paprika

1 tsp chili powder

¼ tsp cayenne pepper

2 cups (63 g) tightly packed spinach

2 tsp (4 g) ground turmeric

½ cup (62 g) shredded vegan cheese of choice (optional, but recommended)

GARNISHES

2 ripe avocados, sliced

Green onion

Fresh cilantro

Hot sauce

Make the potatoes: Preheat the oven to 450°F (230°C).

Place the cubed potatoes on a baking sheet, then add the coconut oil, garlic powder, cumin, smoked paprika, salt and pepper. Toss well to evenly coat, then lay out in a single layer. Roast in the oven, for 22 to 27 minutes, tossing once halfway through the roasting time, until fork-tender and golden brown. Remove from the oven and set aside.

While the potatoes roast, make the scramble: Drain and rinse the tofu, then wrap the bricks in clean dish towels. Place heavy objects, such as books or a cast-iron skillet, on top to help remove as much water as possible. Let sit for 10 minutes.

In a large skillet, preferably cast iron, melt the coconut oil over medium-high heat. Once hot, add the red onion and sauté, stirring occasionally, for 7 minutes. Season generously with salt and black pepper.

Add the bell pepper and cook for 3 to 5 minutes to soften. Add the garlic, paprika, chili powder and cayenne. Cook, stirring well, for 1 minute to evenly coat the vegetables. Add the spinach and cook, stirring constantly, for 1 to 2 minutes, to slightly wilt.

Using your hands, crumble the tofu into small bite-size pieces over the skillet. Add the turmeric and cook, stirring constantly, for 5 to 7 minutes, or until everything is combined and the tofu is yellow. If using the vegan cheese, add it 2 to 3 minutes before the scramble is done cooking, to melt. Season with salt and pepper to taste.

Divide the potatoes and scramble equally among 4 serving bowls and top with the avocado, green onion, cilantro and hot sauce.

If making ahead of time, mix everything together as directed, except leave off the avocado until ready to serve. Keep in an airtight container in the fridge for up to a week.

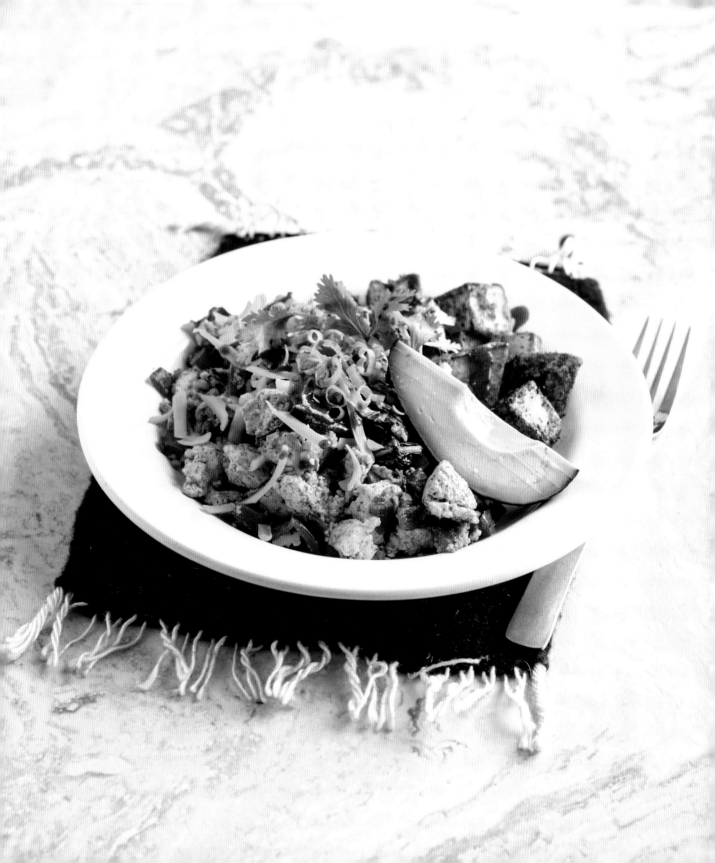

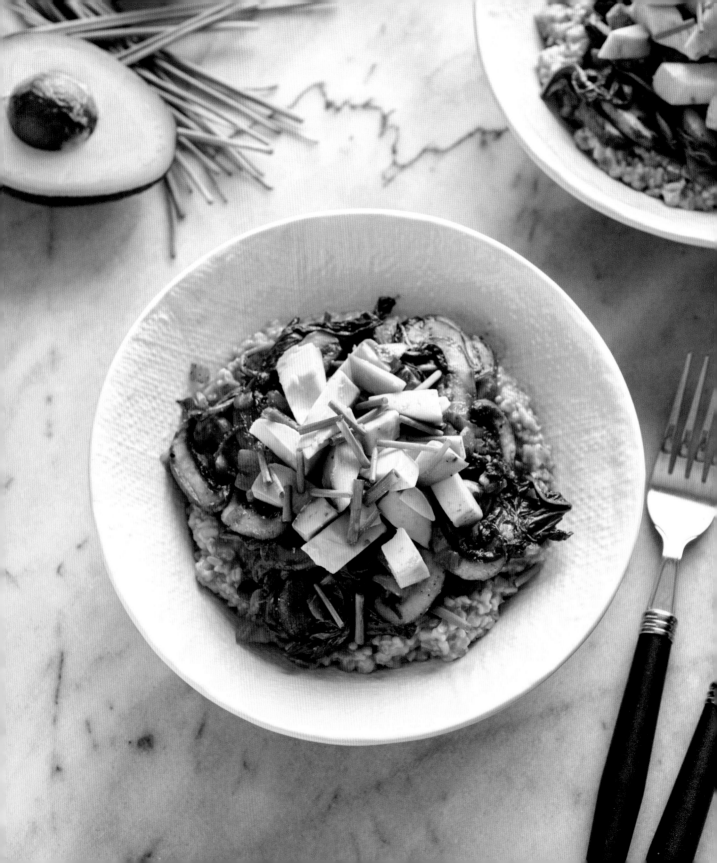

Savory Mushroom Oatmeal

*I am a savory girl through and through, and this oatmeal is what my breakfast dreams
are made of. The creamy oatmeal is super flavorful because it is made with vegetable broth,
and the combination of spinach and mushrooms is hard to beat. For it having so
few ingredients, you will be surprised with how delicious this is!*

SERVES 4

OATS

6 cups (1.4 L) vegetable broth

1½ cups (120 g) steel-cut oats

VEGETABLES

1 tbsp (14 g) coconut oil

1 cup (150 g) diced yellow onion

Salt and freshly ground black pepper

5 cups (350 g) thinly sliced cremini
mushrooms

5½ cups (175 g) tightly packed
spinach

2 tsp (6 g) garlic powder

2 tbsp (30 ml) tamari or soy sauce

GARNISHES

Chopped fresh chives

1 avocado, peeled, pitted and diced

Make the oats: In a medium-sized soup pot, bring the vegetable broth to a boil. Slowly stir in the oats and cook for 5 minutes, or until they begin to thicken. Lower the heat to a simmer and cook, uncovered, for about 30 minutes, stirring occasionally.

Meanwhile, make the vegetables: In a large skillet, melt the coconut oil over medium heat. Once hot, add the onion and season generously with salt and pepper. Cook for 5 minutes, then add the mushrooms and cook, stirring occasionally, for 7 to 9 minutes, or until cooked through. Add the spinach and cook, stirring, until wilted. Turn off the heat, add the garlic powder and tamari and stir to combine. Set aside.

Divide the oats equally among 4 serving bowls and top each with the mushroom mixture. Garnish with chives and avocado and serve.

If making ahead of time, prepare everything as directed, except save the avocado until serving. Store the oatmeal in an airtight container in the fridge until ready to serve. To reheat, use a microwave or, alternatively, a saucepan with a little vegetable broth to prevent sticking.

Caramelized Banana Smoothie Bowl

Although this is in the breakfast section, it could absolutely pass for dessert. And it is anything but a boring smoothie bowl! The caramelized bananas are delectable paired with the banana nice cream that has peanut butter notes popping through every bite. The date caramel, topped with hemp seeds, peanuts and coconut flakes, makes it extra special! My boyfriend always has the most satisfied smile on his face when I make this!

SERVES 2

DATE CARAMEL

½ cup (88 g) pitted Medjool dates

¼ cup (85 g) honey or coconut nectar (see Note)

¼ cup (60 ml) full-fat coconut milk, plus more if needed

½ tsp vanilla extract

Pinch of pink salt

CARAMELIZED BANANAS

Melted coconut oil, for plate

2 ripe bananas

¼ cup (56 g) granulated coconut sugar or (60 g) brown sugar

1 tbsp (14 g) vegan butter, plus more to prevent sticking

BANANA NICE CREAM

½ cup (120 ml) almond milk

6 frozen bananas, sliced into small disks

2 tbsp (32 g) smooth peanut butter

GARNISHES

Peanuts

Hemp seeds

Coconut flakes

Make the date caramel: In a high-speed blender, combine the dates, honey, coconut milk, vanilla extract and salt and blend until smooth and creamy. You can adjust the consistency by adding more coconut milk if it's too thick or you prefer a thinner caramel.

Make the caramelized bananas: Lightly oil a large plate and set aside. Slice the bananas on the diagonal into thick slices. Put the coconut sugar on a separate plate and roll the banana slices in the sugar until evenly coated. In a skillet, melt the vegan butter over medium-low heat. Once hot, add the sliced bananas and cook for 5 to 7 minutes per side, being mindful not to let them burn—if you smell or see them browning, be sure to flip to the other side. Once both sides have been browned, transfer them to the oiled plate. Set aside and let cool for 10 minutes.

When the caramelized bananas have cooled, make the nice cream: In a high-speed blender, combine the almond milk, frozen bananas and peanut butter and blend until smooth, stopping to scrape down the sides or use the tamper, if needed.

To serve, divide up the banana nice cream between 2 bowls and top with the caramelized bananas and date caramel. Garnish with peanuts, hemp seeds and coconut flakes. Serve immediately.

Note: *I do not recommend maple syrup in this recipe. You can use brown rice syrup if you do not have honey or coconut nectar.*

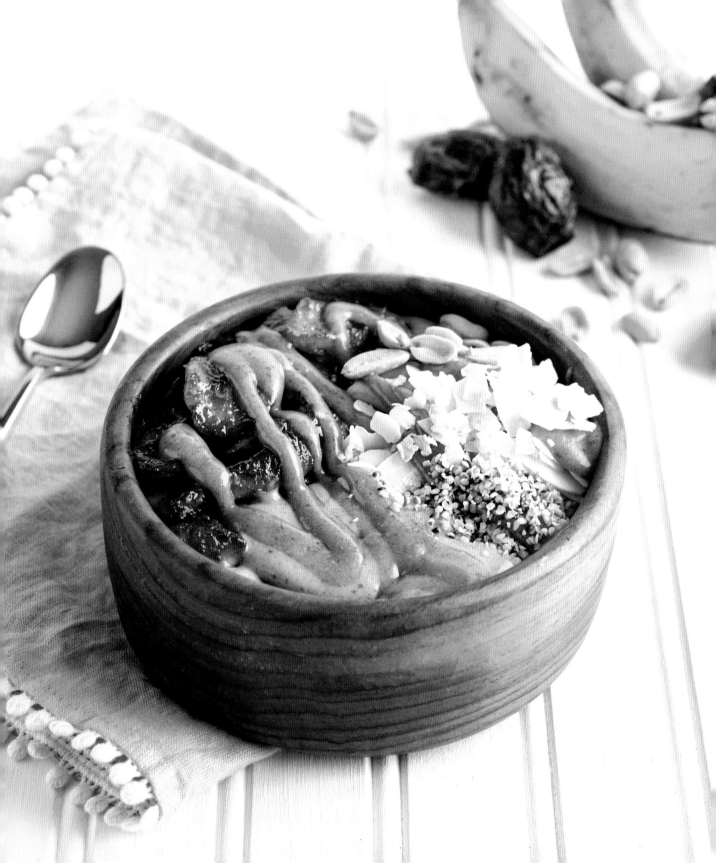

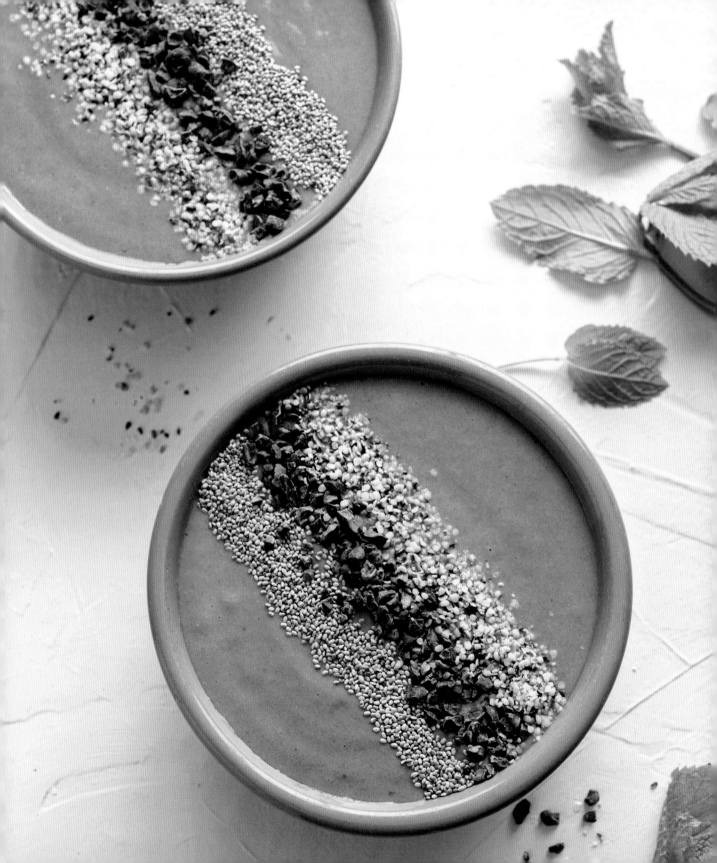

Mint Chip Smoothie Bowl

Have you ever added cauliflower to your smoothies? It's surprisingly awesome because you can't taste it once it's blended and it's a great way for you to still enjoy a delicious smoothie full of fiber and nutrients! The cauliflower makes it nice and thick, while the protein powder, mint and cacao make it delicious. If you are a mint chip fan, you will surely enjoy this!

SMOOTHIE

4 cups (400 g) chopped, steamed, then frozen cauliflower florets (½" [1.2-cm] pieces) (see Note)

1 scoop chocolate protein powder

6 to 8 fresh mint leaves

2 tsp (3 g) cacao powder

2 tsp (10 ml) pure maple syrup

3 cups (710 ml) sweetened almond milk

GARNISHES

Hemp seeds

Chia seeds

Cacao nibs

In a high-speed blender, combine the frozen cauliflower, protein powder, mint leaves, cacao powder, maple syrup and almond milk. Blend on high speed until smooth. Transfer to 2 serving bowls and top with hemp seeds, chia seeds and cacao nibs.

Note: *Steam the cauliflower florets before freezing to make the smoothie easier to digest and provide a creamier texture.*

Chocolate Peanut Butter Smoothie Bowl

This smoothie is so delicious, you'd never guess it's made with nutrient-dense cauliflower! The combination of chocolate and peanut butter is a classic for a reason—it's so good. With both the protein powder and peanut butter, this smoothie bowl is also very filling and great postworkout on a warm day. Garnished with some epic toppings and you have yourself a dream in a bowl.

SERVES 2

SMOOTHIE

4 cups (400 g) chopped, steamed, then frozen cauliflower florets (½" [1.2-cm] pieces) (see Note)

1 scoop chocolate protein powder

3 tbsp (32 g) peanut butter

2 tsp (3 g) cacao powder

3 cups (710 ml) sweetened almond milk

2 tsp (10 ml) honey

GARNISHES

Crushed peanuts

Peanut butter

Honey

Cacao nibs

In a high-speed blender, combine the cauliflower, chocolate protein powder, peanut butter, cacao powder, almond milk and honey. Blend on high speed until smooth, stopping to scrape down the sides, if needed.

Transfer to 2 bowls and top with crushed peanuts, peanut butter, honey and cacao nibs.

Note: Steam the cauliflower florets before freezing to make the smoothie easier to digest and provide a creamier texture.

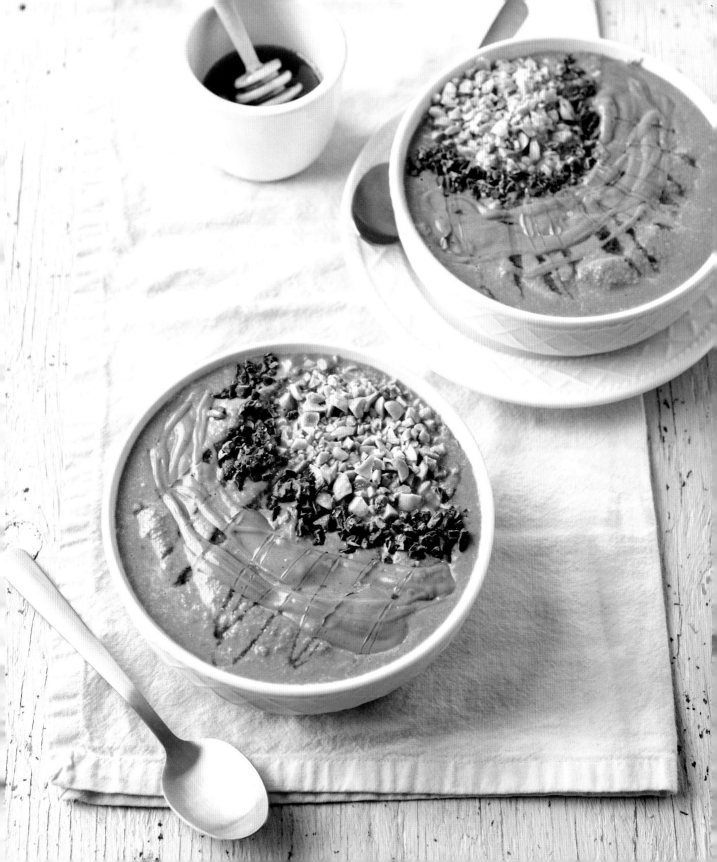

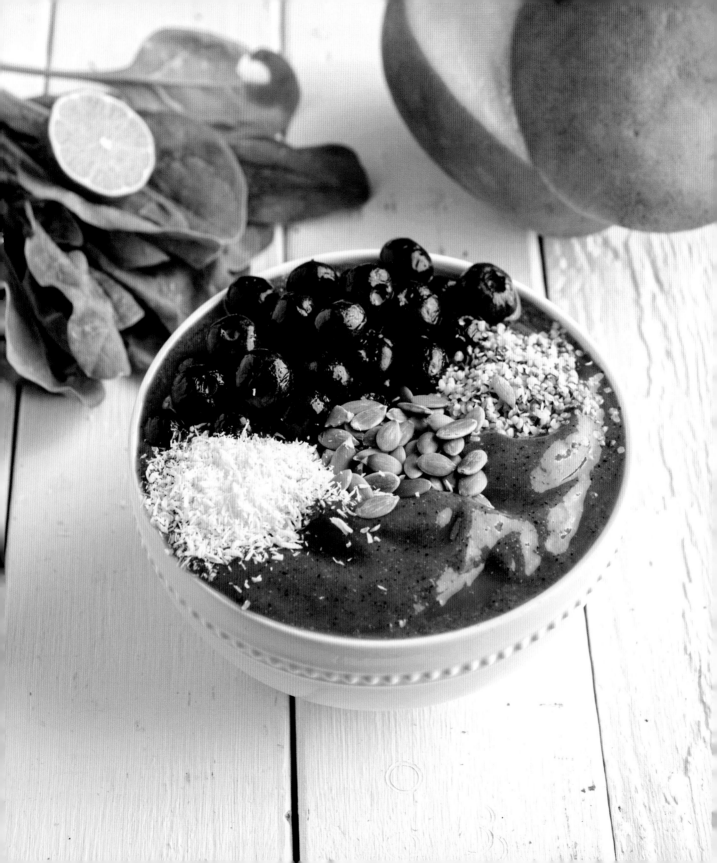

Mango & Bluebs Smoothie Bowl

See! I like fruit in smoothies, too, and this is one of my favorites to enjoy in the summer after a sweaty hike or yoga class. It's refreshingly sweet from the mango, blueberries and banana, and supertangy from the lime juice, which I totally love. You will likely be a big fan, too!

SERVES 2

SMOOTHIE

1 banana, peeled and frozen

3 cups (495 g) frozen mango cubes

1 cup (155 g) frozen blueberries

1 cup (32 g) tightly packed spinach leaves

1½ cups (355 ml) unsweetened almond milk

2 tbsp (30 ml) fresh lime juice

GARNISHES

Shredded coconut

Hemp seeds

Pumpkin seeds

Frozen blueberries

In a high-powered blender, combine the banana, mango, blueberries, spinach, almond milk and lime juice. Blend on high speed until smooth.

Transfer to 2 serving bowls and top with the shredded coconut, hemp seeds, pumpkin seeds and frozen blueberries.

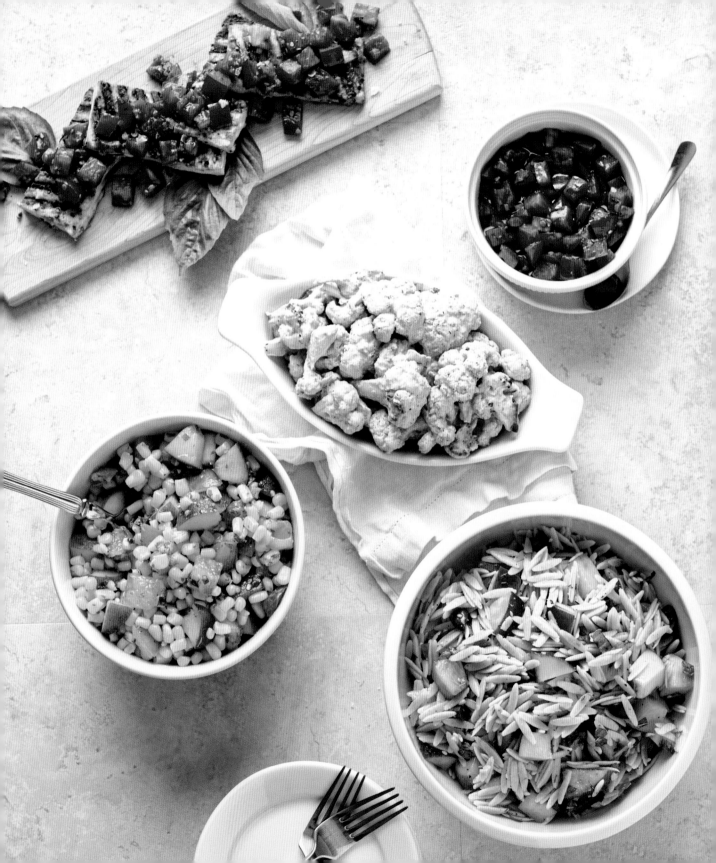

Simply Delicious Sides

I find that, whenever side dishes are involved, often lots of people are involved! Which is something I love about food: how it has the power to bring people together and become a part of some of our most cherished memories. Some of my favorite crowd-pleasing sides from this book are the Minty Stone Fruit Salad (page 136, perfect for summer barbecues or picnics), Tropical Vegan Ceviche (page 132, great for pool parties or birthday parties), Curried Cauliflower & Sorghum (page 143, great for potlucks) and Cilantro-Tahini Broccoli (page 128, ideal for dinner parties).

In addition to being great sides on their own, there are several other fun ways to incorporate these recipes. For topping toast, including avocado toast or as a bruschetta topping, try the Spicy Summer Salad (page 139), Passion Fruit, Peach & Avocado Party (page 147) or the Marinated Basil Tomatoes (page 144). These would also be delicious mixed with some orzo or bow-tie pasta, or to accompany a grilled protein of choice (such as tofu or fish, if you eat it) and even with mixed greens to transform it into a salad. Just a few ideas to try, but feel free to get creative and dream up new ways to utilize these vibrant plant-based sides!

Cilantro-Tahini Broccoli

Tahini has such a distinct flavor on its own. It's not like other nut or seed butters for example peanut butter or sunflower seed butter; it's very bitter and doesn't taste that great. However, when combined with a few other ingredients, it is so delightful. This sauce hits all the notes—savory, bitter, salty, sour and sweet. It pairs perfectly with broccoli, which is so delicious when roasted, because roasting brings out the natural sweetness while keeping some of the crunch!

───────── SERVES 4 AS A SIDE ─────────

BROCCOLI

8 cups (568 g) chopped broccoli florets

2 tbsp (30 ml) melted coconut oil

Salt and freshly ground black pepper

CILANTRO TAHINI SAUCE

⅓ cup (13 g) finely chopped fresh cilantro, plus more for garnish (optional)

¼ cup (60 ml) avocado oil

3 tbsp (45 ml) fresh lime juice

1½ tbsp (23 ml) apple cider vinegar

2 tbsp (30 g) tahini

1 tsp pure maple syrup

1 clove garlic, grated (preferred) or minced

Salt and freshly ground black pepper

Preheat the oven to 450°F (230°C).

Make the broccoli: Place the broccoli on a baking sheet and add the coconut oil. Add salt and pepper to taste, then toss well. Spread into a single layer and roast in the oven for 15 to 20 minutes, or until the edges are turning brown and getting crispy. Transfer to a large serving bowl.

Make the sauce: In a small bowl, vigorously whisk together the cilantro, avocado oil, lime juice, vinegar, tahini, maple syrup, garlic and salt and pepper to taste. Pour the sauce over the broccoli and mix well. Serve immediately, topping with more cilantro, if desired.

This is great for meal prep, so if making ahead of time, store in an airtight container in the fridge for up to a week!

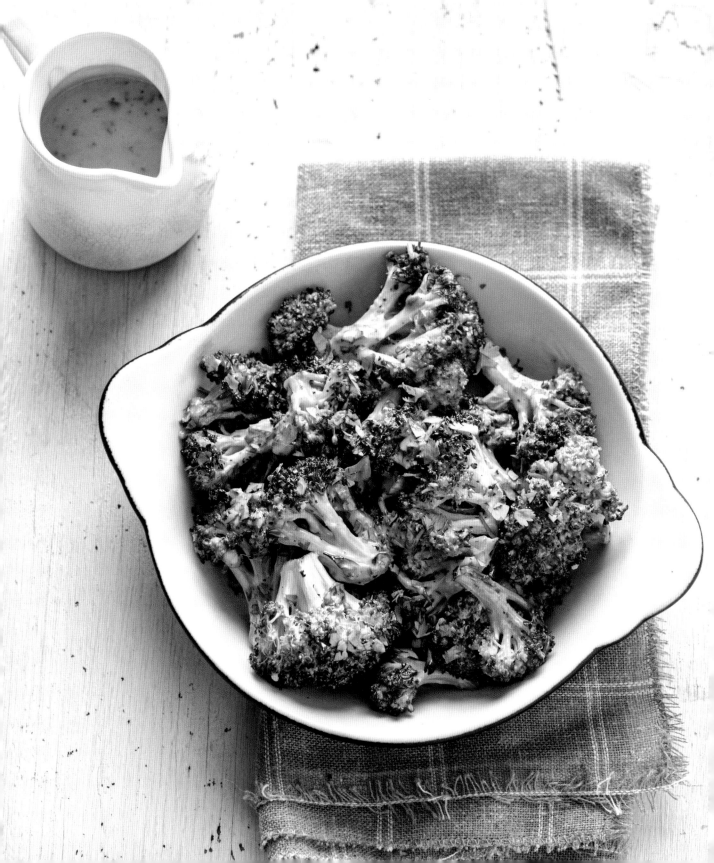

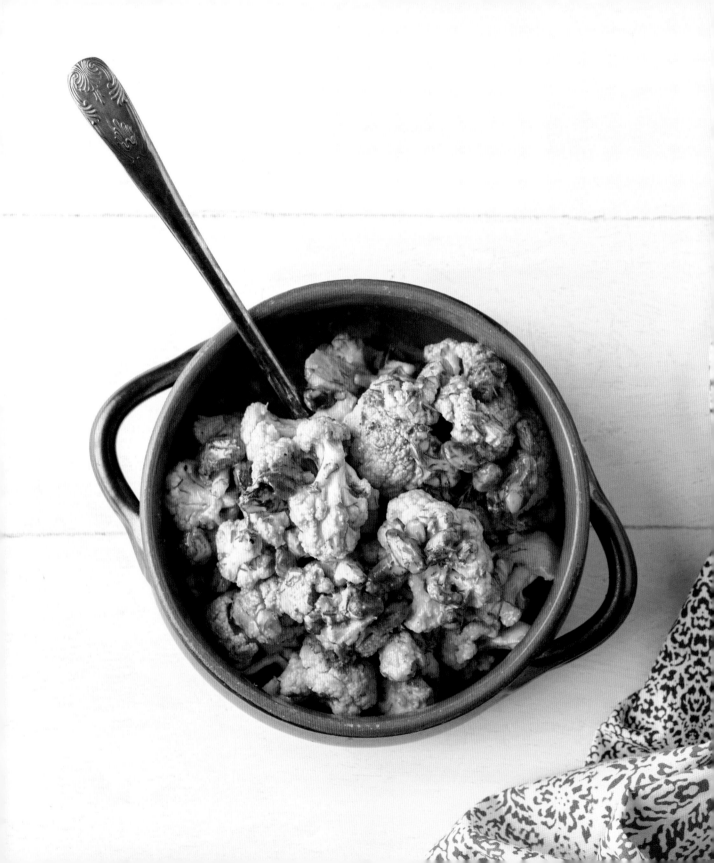

Harissa-Tahini Cauliflower

This cauliflower dish is easily one of my favorites because it's easy to make but feels decadent. The spicy harissa is calm at first and intensifies as you chew, but it is balanced out by the bitter tahini and sour lemon, giving it a delicious flavor and mouthfeel. The pistachios add crunch, the raisins bring sweetness and the herbs keep it feeling fresh!

--- SERVES 2 AS A SIDE ---

HARISSA TAHINI SAUCE

¼ cup (60 g) tahini

⅓ cup (80 ml) water

1 tbsp (15 ml) fresh lemon juice

2 tsp (10 g) harissa paste

1 tsp pure maple syrup

Salt

CAULIFLOWER

1 large head cauliflower, cut into bite-size florets

2 tbsp (30 ml) melted coconut oil

Salt

2 tbsp (5 g) chopped fresh mint

1½ tbsp (6 g) chopped fresh dill

¼ cup (31 g) pistachios

3 tbsp (27 g) golden raisins

Freshly ground black pepper

Preheat the oven to 450°F (230°C).

Make the sauce: In a small bowl, whisk together the tahini, water, lemon juice, harissa and maple syrup. Add salt to taste and set aside.

Make the cauliflower: Lay out the cauliflower florets on a baking sheet and add the coconut oil and a generous pinch of salt. Mix well so the cauliflower is evenly coated with the oil. Spread out in an even layer and roast in the oven for 15 to 25 minutes, or until golden brown on 1 side and the edges are getting crispy.

Remove from the oven and let cool for 10 minutes. Then, transfer to a medium-sized serving bowl and top with the sauce, mint, dill, pistachios, raisins and salt and pepper to taste. Mix well and serve!

This is also great for meal prep, so if making ahead of time, store in an airtight container in the fridge for up to a week!

Tropical Vegan Ceviche

This is absolutely a dreamy combination of ingredients. If Tulum, Mexico, were a recipe, it would be this. It's sweet, spicy, tangy and salty and just screams beachy vibes. Eat it with a fork, with chips or put it on top of grilled tofu, or salmon or chicken if you are a meat eater, or mix it in with the Energizing Sweet Potato & Greens Salad (page 54), as it goes so well with the coconut bacon in that recipe. You will love this colorful, flavorful dish!

SERVES 6 AS A SIDE

---

1 cup (175 g) diced mango (½" [1.2-cm] cubes)

1 cup (175 g) diced papaya (½" [1.2-cm] cubes)

1 cup (155 g) diced pineapple (½" [1.2-cm] cubes)

1 cup (130 g) diced jicama (½" [1.2-cm] cubes)

1 cup (146 g) diced hearts of palm (½" [1.2-cm] cubes)

1 cup (135 g) diced English cucumber

1 cup (40 g) loosely packed chopped fresh cilantro

1 cup (150 g) diced red onion

½ cup (50 g) sliced green onion

½ cup (120 ml) fresh lime juice

Zest of 4 limes

2 tsp (6 g) chili powder

¼ tsp cayenne pepper

Salt and freshly ground black pepper

TO SERVE

Avocado

Vegan tortilla chips

In a medium-sized bowl, combine the mango, papaya, pineapple, jicama, hearts of palm, cucumber, cilantro, red onion, green onion, lime juice and zest, chili powder and cayenne pepper. Mix well and then season to taste with salt and black pepper. Let marinate in the fridge for 15 minutes, stirring every 5 minutes, before serving.

When ready to serve, mix in some avocado cubes to the ceviche and serve with chips.

This is best served fresh, but can be made 2 to 3 hours ahead of time if needed. Store in an airtight container in the fridge, reserving the avocado and chips until ready to serve.

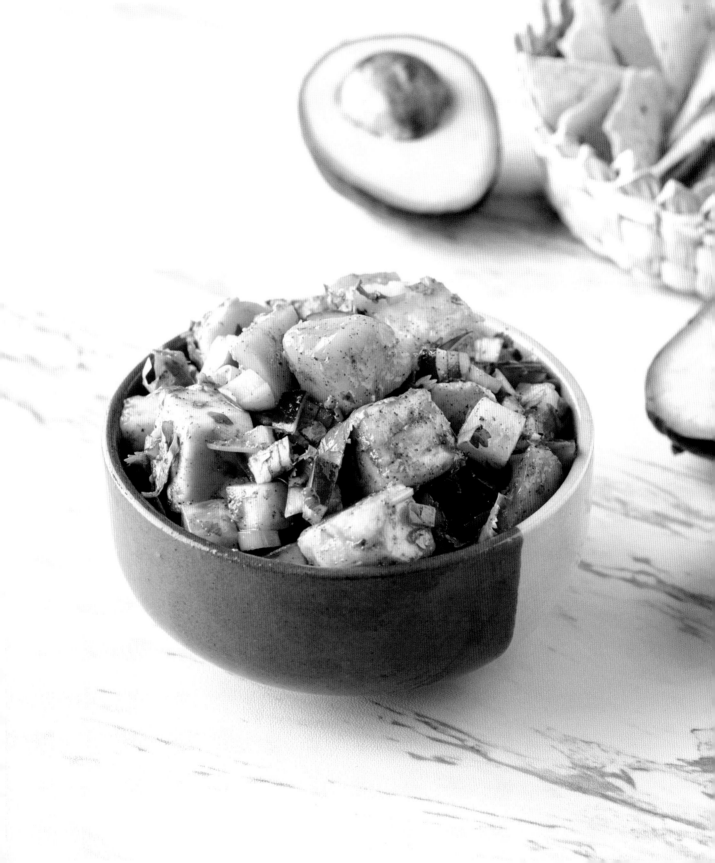

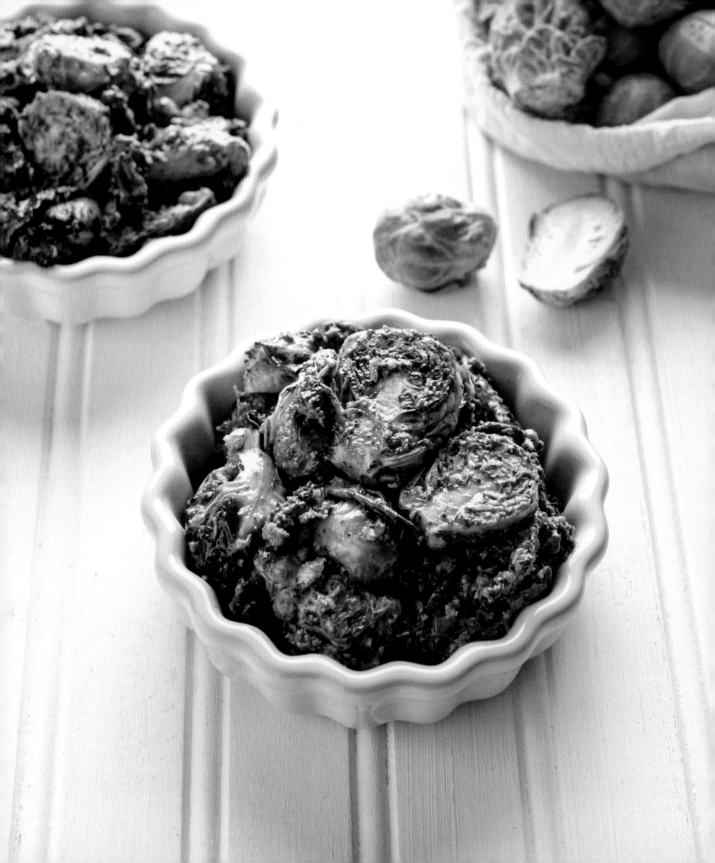

Basil Pesto Brussels Sprouts

This is one of my go-tos if I am making something for a potluck when Brussels sprouts are in season. The bright and subtly sweet pesto is balanced out perfectly by the bitter and subtly sweet roasted veggie. And the sun-dried tomatoes add texture and flavor that really make the dish feel complete.

SERVES 4 AS A SIDE

BRUSSELS SPROUTS

8 cups (704 g) trimmed and halved Brussels sprouts

2 tbsp (28 g) coconut oil

Salt and freshly ground black pepper

1 cup (110 g) chopped oil-packed sun-dried tomatoes

BASIL PESTO

¼ cup (34 g) pine nuts

2 cloves garlic

1 tbsp (8 g) nutritional yeast

3 cups (120 g) lightly packed fresh basil leaves

Juice of 1 lemon

½ tsp salt

¼ cup (60 ml) olive oil

Preheat the oven to 450°F (230°C).

Lay out the Brussels sprouts in a single layer on 1 or 2 baking sheets. Coat evenly with the oil and season with salt and black pepper to taste. Mix well. Roast in the oven for 12 to 17 minutes, or until crispy and browned on 1 side.

Meanwhile, make the pesto: In a food processor, combine the pine nuts, garlic, nutritional yeast, basil leaves, lemon juice and salt and pulse in 3-second bursts for a total of 30 to 45 seconds, or until everything is finely diced but not turned into a paste. Then, with the processor on low speed, slowly drizzle in the olive oil through the center of the lid until a thick, slight chunky paste is formed. Set aside.

Once the Brussels sprouts are done, transfer them to a large bowl with the sun-dried tomatoes and pesto. Mix well to evenly coat and serve.

If making ahead, simply store in the refrigerator in an airtight container for up to a week.

Minty Stone Fruit Salad

Juicy sweet peaches, savory salty olives, herbaceous bright mint? That's a combination that would make anyone's taste buds happy. Mixed with orzo pasta and spiced up with some za'atar, this may just be your new favorite pasta salad!

SERVES 6 AS A SIDE

LEMON VINAIGRETTE

½ cup (120 ml) olive oil

¼ cup (60 ml) fresh lemon juice

1 tsp garlic powder

Salt and freshly ground black pepper

PASTA

1 lb (455 g) orzo pasta

1 cup (170 g) diced nectarine
(½" [1.2-cm] cubes)

1 cup (170 g) diced peach (½" [1.2-cm] cubes)

1 cup (100 g) pitted and roughly chopped Kalamata olives

¼ cup (11 g) tightly packed finely chopped fresh mint

1 tbsp (8 g) za'atar

Make the vinaigrette: In a small bowl, vigorously whisk together the olive oil, lemon juice, garlic powder and salt and pepper to taste. Set aside.

Make the pasta: Bring a medium-sized pot of salted water to a boil. Add the orzo and cooking according to the package instructions. Drain and rinse with cold water until the pasta is cool.

Transfer the pasta to a serving bowl and add the nectarine, peach, olives, mint, za'atar and vinaigrette. Mix well to combine and serve.

This is great for meal prep, so if making ahead of time, store in an airtight container in the fridge for up to a week!

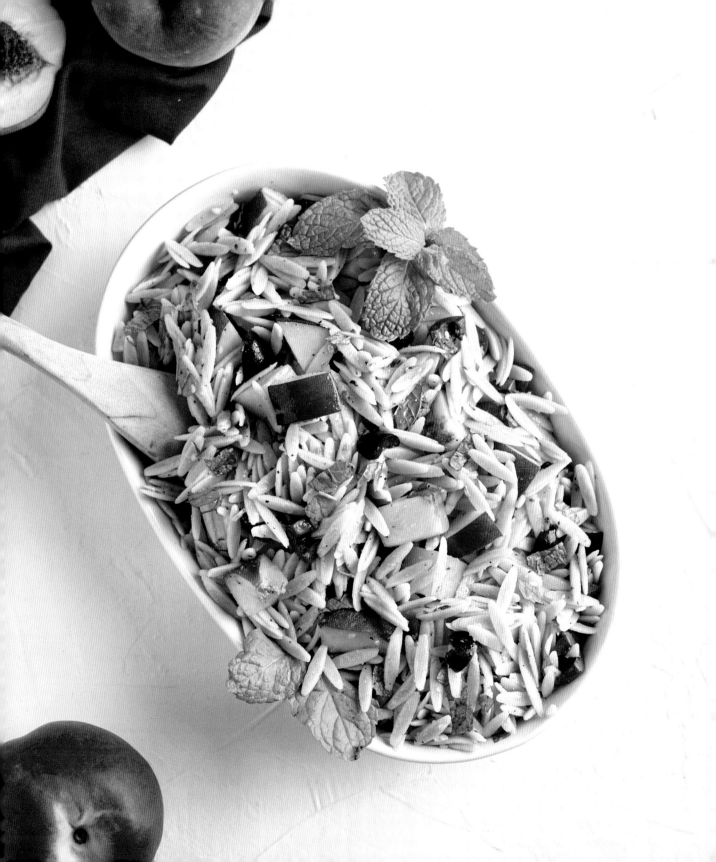

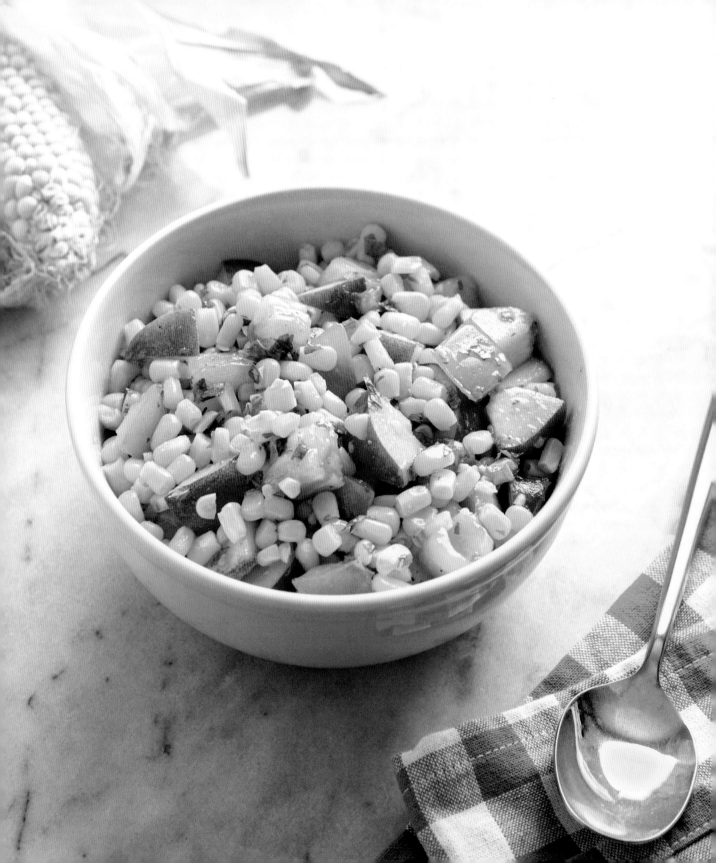

Spicy Summer Salad

This recipe ends up feeling like a lazy-fancy salsa or fruit salad and it screams "summer barbecue." It pairs perfectly with grilled tofu, or even mozzarella slices, Cotija cheese or chicken if you are a dairy or meat eater. And if you are feeling fancy, add some toasted pepitas! It's also great on its own. The chili vinaigrette really shines next to the sweet corn, peaches and heirlooms. The bright mint adds a little something extra that ties it all together.

--- SERVES 6 AS A SIDE ---

CHILI VINAIGRETTE

½ cup (120 ml) grapeseed or avocado oil

1 tsp crushed red pepper flakes

⅛ tsp cayenne pepper

½ tsp garlic powder

¼ cup (60 ml) fresh lime juice

Salt and freshly ground black pepper

SALAD

3 cups (510 g) diced peach (½" [1.2-cm] cubes)

2½ cups (375 g) corn kernels, cut fresh from the cob

2 cups (360 g) diced heirloom tomato (½" [1.2-cm] cubes)

¼ cup (11 g) tightly packed finely chopped fresh mint

¼ cup (11 g) tightly packed chopped cilantro

Make the dressing: In a small bowl, combine the oil, red pepper flakes and cayenne. Let marinate for 20 minutes. Then, whisk in the garlic powder, lime juice and salt and pepper to taste.

Make the salad: In a serving bowl, combine the peach, corn, tomato, mint, cilantro and dressing. Mix well and serve.

If making ahead of time, prepare the salad and keep separately from the dressing in an airtight container in the fridge until serving. Keeps well for up to 3 days.

Roasted Cauliflower with Herb Cream

At this point in the book, it is probably no surprise that I am a big fan of using cashews to make sauce and add herbs to almost everything I make. And you know what they say: If it ain't broke, don't fix it. So keeping on with my love for creamy cashews and fresh herbs, I bring you this elevated take on roasted cauliflower. I am pretty sure you will love it as much as I do! The sauce coats each floret in creamy green heaven.

———————— SERVES 4 AS A SIDE ————————

FRESH HERB CREAM

½ cup (70 g) raw cashews, soaked in very hot water for 12 minutes (see Note)

¼ cup (60 ml) water

2 tbsp (30 ml) fresh lemon juice

¼ cup (11 g) tightly packed fresh basil or cilantro leaves

2 tbsp (8 g) fresh dill

¼ tsp salt

Freshly ground black pepper

CAULIFLOWER

8 cups (800 g) chopped cauliflower florets

2 tbsp (30 ml) melted coconut oil

Salt and freshly ground black pepper

Preheat the oven to 450°F (230°C).

Make the herb cream: Drain and rinse the cashews, then place them in a blender. Add the fresh water, lemon juice, basil, dill, salt and pepper to taste. Blend on high speed until smooth, stopping to scrape down the sides or add additional water as needed to reach your desired consistency. Set aside.

Make the cauliflower: Lay out the cauliflower in a single layer on 1 or 2 baking sheets. Coat evenly with the coconut oil and salt and pepper to taste. Roast in the oven for 13 to 20 minutes, or until golden brown and cooked through.

Transfer the cauliflower to a serving bowl and add the herb cream. Mix well and serve.

If making ahead, simply store in the refrigerator in an airtight container for up to a week.

Note: *If you do not have a high-speed blender, soak your cashews for an hour or overnight, to protect your blender.*

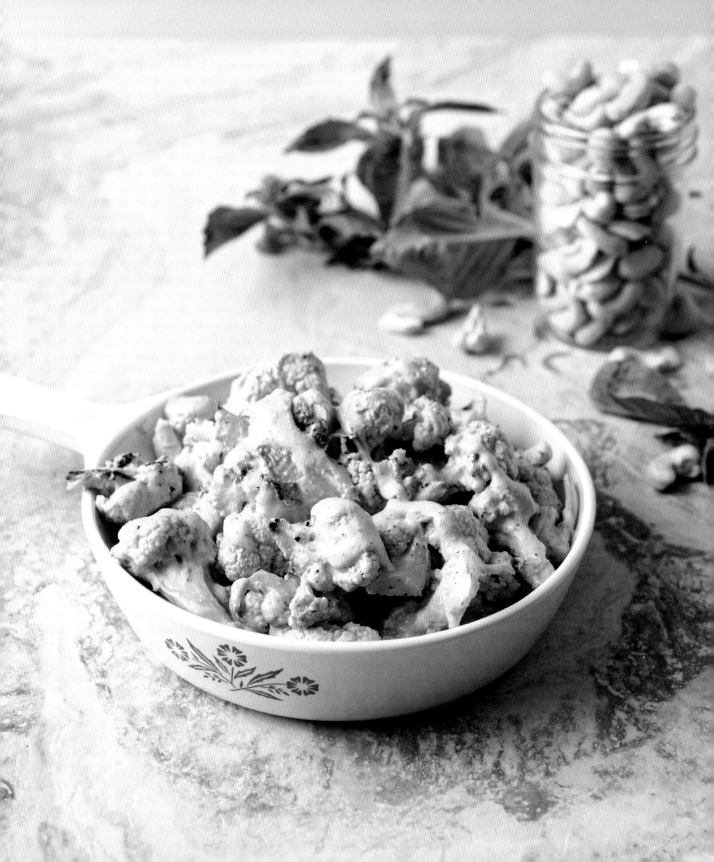

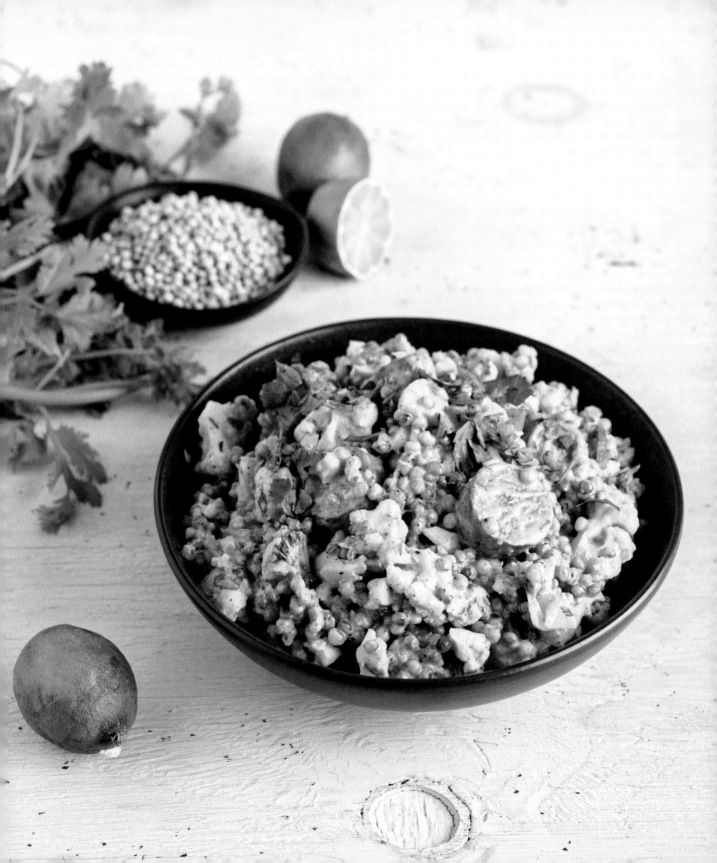

Curried Cauliflower & Sorghum

Oh, this side salad! It is inspired by a side at one of my favorite sandwich chains in Los Angeles, called Mendocino Farms. I wanted to use a hearty, more nutrient-dense grain in my version and sorghum fit the bill perfectly. It's full of fiber, protein, carbs and a chewy texture with a great bite. The curried mayo is insanely good—spiced perfectly and totally pops from the lime juice. The cilantro, cauliflower and carrots add some additional nutrients, texture and color. This is so perfect for barbecues, pool parties, potlucks, picnics and lunches.

–––––––––––––––––––– SERVES 6 AS A SIDE ––––––––––––––––––––

2 cups (400 g) whole-grain sorghum

6 cups (1.4 L) vegetable broth or water

1 medium-sized head cauliflower, chopped into ½" (1.2-cm) florets

4 carrots, chopped into bite-size pieces

2 tbsp (30 ml) avocado oil

½ cup (21 g) tightly packed chopped fresh cilantro

Salt and freshly ground black pepper

SAUCE

1 cup (225 g) vegan mayonnaise

2 tbsp (30 ml) fresh lime juice

1 tbsp (15 ml) pure maple syrup

1 tbsp (6 g) curry powder

Salt and freshly ground black pepper

Preheat the oven to 450°F (230°C).

In a medium-sized lidded pot, combine the sorghum and vegetable broth and bring to a boil. Cover and lower the heat to a simmer. Cook for 50 to 60 minutes, or until the liquid is absorbed and the sorghum is cooked through. Drain and rinse with cold water.

Meanwhile, lay out the cauliflower and carrots on a baking sheet and cover with the avocado oil. Toss to coat well and then roast in the oven for 12 to 15 minutes, or until soft. Remove from the oven and set aside.

Make the sauce: In a small bowl, combine the mayo, lime juice, maple syrup, curry powder and salt and pepper to taste. Mix well.

In a large serving bowl, combine the sorghum, cauliflower, carrots, cilantro and the sauce. Add salt and pepper to taste. Mix well and serve.

This is great for meal prep, so if making ahead of time, store in an airtight container in the fridge for up to a week!

Marinated Basil Tomatoes

This is a classic combination for bruschetta topping or for a Caprese salad, but I am a huge fan of putting it on avocado toast or mixing it in with pasta. When tomatoes and basil are at their peak in summer, this is hard to beat.

--- SERVES 4 AS A SIDE ---

BASIL & BALSAMIC VINAIGRETTE

⅓ cup (80 ml) olive oil

2 tbsp (30 ml) balsamic vinegar

2 tbsp (6 g) tightly packed finely chopped fresh basil

2 cloves garlic, minced

Salt and freshly ground black pepper

TOMATOES

3 cups (540 g) diced Roma or cherry tomatoes

Make the vinaigrette: In a medium-sized bowl, whisk together the oil, vinegar, basil and garlic. Add salt and pepper to taste.

Add the tomatoes to the vinaigrette and mix well to combine. Let marinate for at least 10 minutes, covered, in the fridge before serving.

If making ahead of time, store in an airtight container in the fridge for up to 3 days.

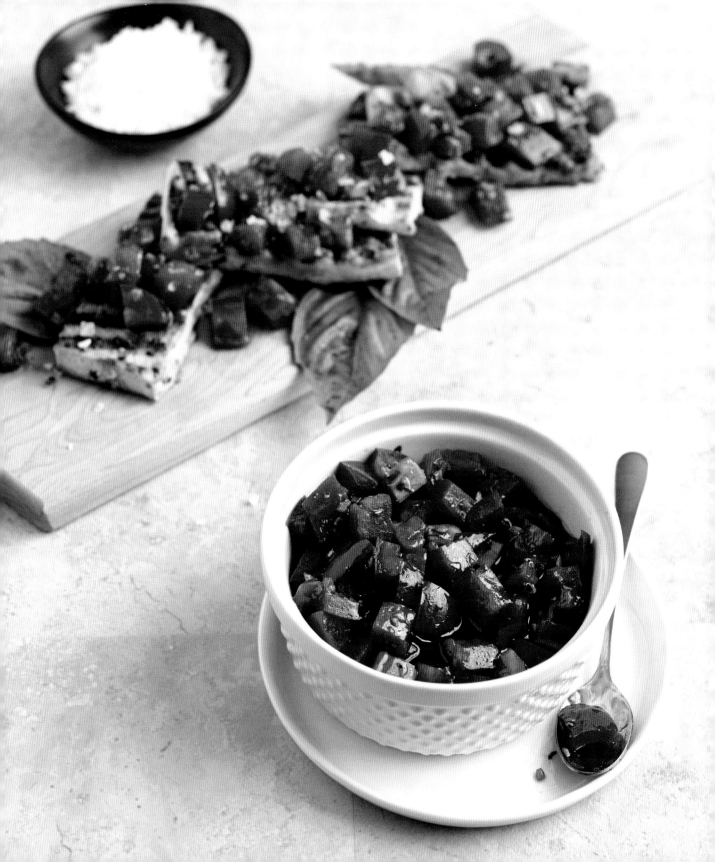

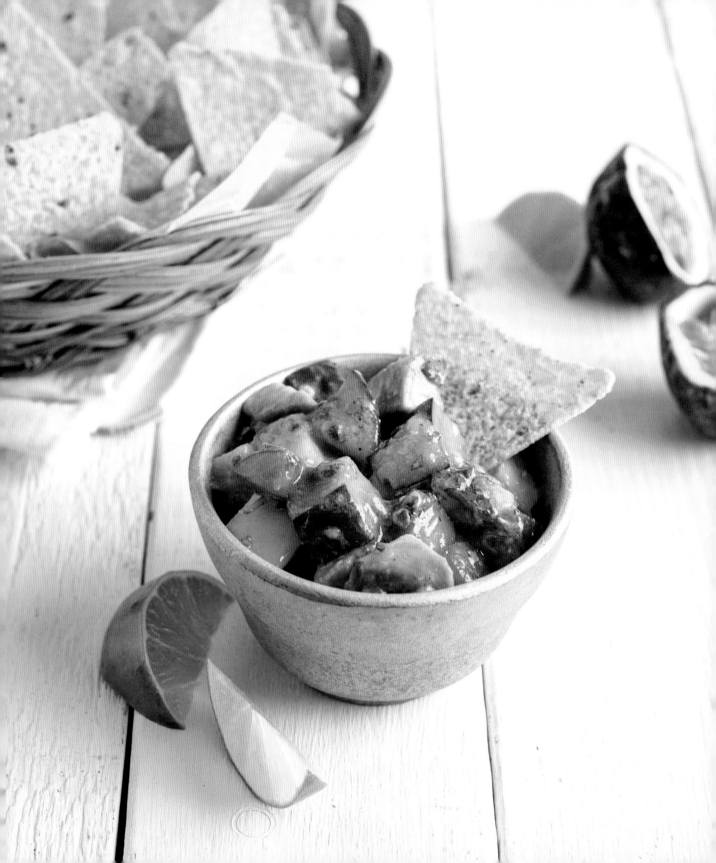

Passion Fruit, Peach & Avocado Party

Passion fruit, avocado and peach are three of my favorite summer produce items from the farmers' markets in Los Angeles, where I live. The tangy passion fruit against the creamy avocado totally pops in your mouth with the sweet juicy peaches. Combining them is simply a dream. This side salad is delicious on its own, with chips, on top of toasts for a fun play on bruschetta as well as on top of grilled tofu or salmon, if you eat meat. You will wow your summer party guests with this one!

SERVES 6 TO 8 AS A SIDE

LIME VINAIGRETTE

½ cup (120 ml) grapeseed or avocado oil

¼ cup (60 ml) fresh lime juice

1 clove garlic, pressed (preferred) or minced

Salt and freshly ground black pepper

BRUSCHETTA

3 cups (510 g) diced peach
(½" [1.2-cm] cubes)

3 cups (438 g) cubed avocado

½ cup (118 g) passion fruit pulp

¼ cup (6 g) tightly packed finely chopped fresh mint

Make the vinaigrette: In a small bowl, whisk together the oil, lime juice, garlic and salt and pepper to taste. Set aside.

In a large bowl, combine the peach, avocado, passion fruit and mint. Top with desired amount of the dressing and mix to combine. Serve.

This dish is best served fresh. Store any remaining dressing in an airtight container in the fridge for up to a week.

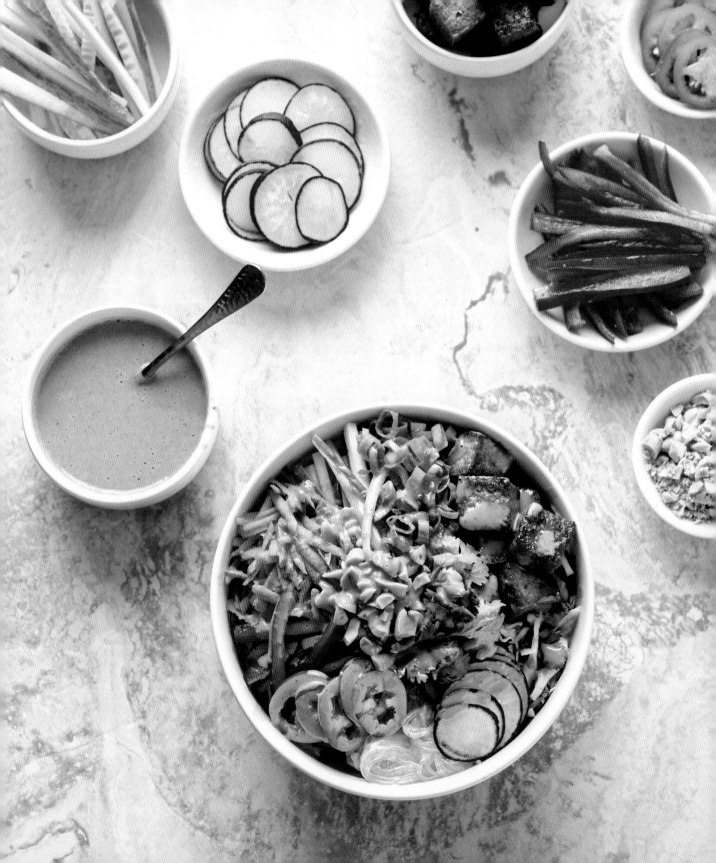

Acknowledgments

Sitting here thinking about who I want to acknowledge feels exciting and at the same time overwhelming, because so many people played a role in this cookbook itself but also in getting me to the point to where this opportunity was possible for me.

Thank you to my parents, who were always supportive of my exploring my love of food. Particularly my dad, who helped me open my first (and only) restaurant and went ahead and self-published my first three e-cookbooks of his own volition, despite my insecure reluctance to share them with the world. He has been my number one fan through all my entrepreneurial ventures.

Thank you to my boyfriend, Brent, who helped do all the dishes without any complaints. And to all my friends who taste-tested countless recipes, including Josephine Dvorak, Jessica Lupo, Meredith and Nick Neath, Dara Siegel, Bree Shook, Hayley Penrose, Christina and Kyle Thompson, Julene McBride, Anna Schott, Jenn Smith, Katherine Kirk, Laura Murphy, Tilita Lutterloh, Michelle Shen and of course, my mom! The cookbook would not be what it is without your help and feedback. I love you all.

Special thanks to Niranjan Khalsa, my two brothers, Justin and Marcus, and Jean Choi, for being awesome supports along the way. To Jackie Sobon, for taking the most amazing photos ever. And to Ashely Rose, Kris Van Genderen, Jamie Vos and Rachel Furman for checking in with my spirit guides to make sure the cookbook was a part of the divine plan as well. To Brandilyn Tebo, for being an amazing life coach who truly changed my life in so many ways.

A massive thank you to Sarah Monroe, my editor, and the entire team at Page Street for believing in me and making this possible.

Last but certainly not least, thank you to every single amazing human being who has ever supported me in any form, my family, friends, those from my Instagram or blog Cara's Kitchen, the podcast Love Your Bod Pod, from my café, Superette and everything in between.

Thank you, sincerely and always grateful,

Xo Cara

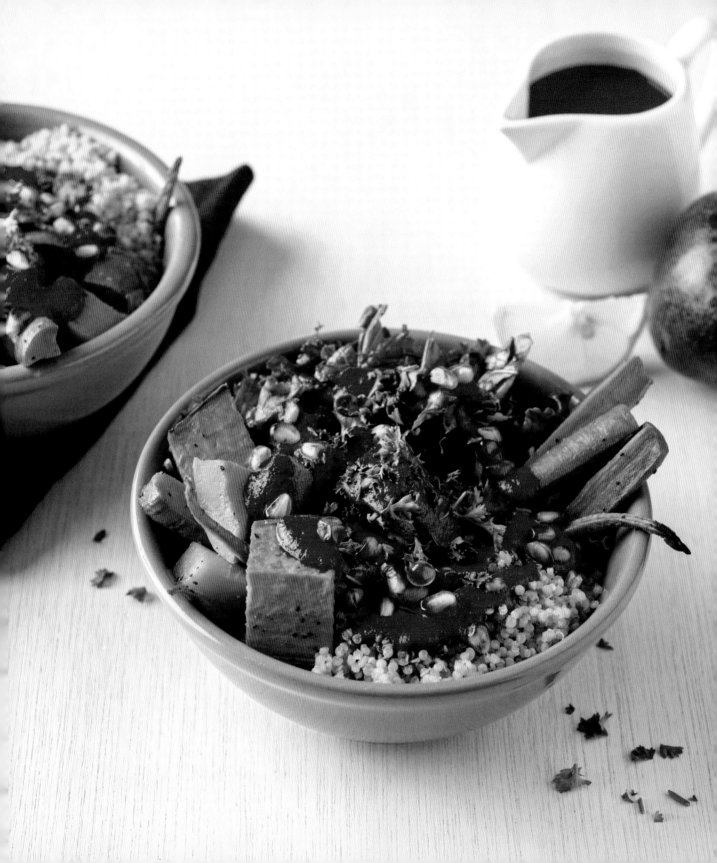

About the Author

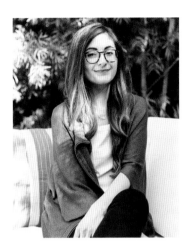

Cara Carin Cifelli is a holistic health coach, author and the voice behind the Love Your Bod Pod podcast. Through her various platforms, she helps people heal their relationships with food and learn to trust their body. Cara is a passionate coach, writer and foodie. When she isn't on Instagram sharing inspiring recipes and tools to help those struggling with disordered eating, she can be found hanging outdoors in sunny Los Angeles, California.

www.caraskitchen.net

Instagram: @caraskitchen

Podcast: Love Your Bod Pod

Twitter: @caracarin

Index